MEDICAL **OFFICE** PROCEDURES

with
Medical Pegboard

5th Edition

MEDICAL OFFICE PROCEDURES

with Medical Pegboard

5th Edition

Eleanor K. Flores, RN, BSN, MEd
Lincoln College of New England
Southington, CT

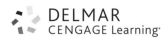

DELMAR
CENGAGE Learning·

Australia · Brazil · Japan · Korea · Mexico · Singapore · Spain · United Kingdom · United States

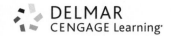
DELMAR
CENGAGE Learning·

Medical Office Procedures with Medical Pegboard, Fifth Edition
Eleanor K. Flores

Vice President, Careers and Computing: Dave Garza

Director of Learning Solutions: Matthew Kane

Executive Editor: Rhonda Dearborn

Managing Editor: Marah Bellegarde

Senior Product Manager: Sarah Prime

Product Manager: Lauren Whalen

Vice President, Marketing: Jennifer Ann Baker

Marketing Director: Wendy E. Mapstone

Senior Marketing Manager: Nancy Bradshaw

Marketing Coordinator: Piper Huntington

Senior Production Director: Wendy A. Troeger

Production Manager: Andrew Crouth

Content Project Manager: Thomas Heffernan

Senior Art Director: Jack Pendleton

For product information and technology assistance, contact us at
Cengage Learning Customer & Sales Support, 1-800-354-9706

For permission to use material from this text or product,
submit all requests online at **www.cengage.com/permissions**.
Further permissions questions can be e-mailed to
permissionrequest@cengage.com

2011 Current Procedural Terminology © 2010 American Medical Association. All Rights Reserved.

Library of Congress Control Number: 2012931962

ISBN-13: 978-1-111-64426-0

ISBN-10: 1-111-64426-8

Delmar
5 Maxwell Drive
Clifton Park, NY 12065-2919
USA

Cengage Learning is a leading provider of customized learning solutions with office locations around the globe, including Singapore, the United Kingdom, Australia, Mexico, Brazil, and Japan. Locate your local office at:
international.cengage.com/region

Cengage Learning products are represented in Canada by Nelson Education, Ltd.

To learn more about Delmar, visit **www.cengage.com/delmar**

Purchase any of our products at your local college store or at our preferred online store **www.cengagebrain.com**

Notice to the Reader

Publisher does not warrant or guarantee any of the products described herein or perform any independent analysis in connection with any of the product information contained herein. Publisher does not assume, and expressly disclaims, any obligation to obtain and include information other than that provided to it by the manufacturer. The reader is expressly warned to consider and adopt all safety precautions that might be indicated by the activities described herein and to avoid all potential hazards. By following the instructions contained herein, the reader willingly assumes all risks in connection with such instructions. The publisher makes no representations or warranties of any kind, including but not limited to, the warranties of fitness for particular purpose or merchantability, nor are any such representations implied with respect to the material set forth herein, and the publisher takes no responsibility with respect to such material. The publisher shall not be liable for any special, consequential, or exemplary damages resulting, in whole or part, from the readers' use of, or reliance upon, this material.

Printed in the United States of America
1 2 3 4 5 6 7 14 13 12

CONTENTS

SECTION 2	**JOBS**	**71**

PREFACE

Combining the fundamental skills of a pegboard system with advances in electronic health records, *Medical Office Procedures with Medical Pegboard* uses hands-on learning to equip you with a solid understanding of the financial activities and events that occur in the medical office. Expanded and completely up to date, it includes the latest advances in key procedures and thoroughly integrates the pegboard into today's medical office environment. The simulation provides hands-on experience with the pegboard system first, laying a solid foundation for learning computerized bookkeeping practices. Using both a pegboard and Medical Office Simulation Software (MOSS) enables you to seamlessly switch between manual and computerized systems, preparing you for real-world practice when you leave the classroom.

After completing *Medical Office Procedures with Medical Pegboard,* you should be able to:

- Record accounts receivable in a pegboard system, including the completion of day sheets, patient ledger cards, receipts, superbills, and daily deposit tickets;
- Record accounts receivable in practice management software, including charges, payments, and adjustments to patient accounts;
- Record both payments from patients and payments from third-party insurance carriers;
- Record accounts payable and payroll entries in a pegboard system, including the drafting of checks, the recording of checks and deposits in the check register, and the tracking of daily account balances;
- Schedule patient appointments and complete an appointment book;
- Prepare a daily patient list so the physician-employer can be informed of patients to be seen and of the nature of their illnesses;
- Complete health insurance forms to be submitted to insurance carriers.

HOW TO USE

Section 1 is a Reference Manual, or informational section. It precedes the simulation and explains all procedures. Section 2 includes all jobs to be performed in the pegboard (or write-it-once) system. Each simulation day ends with closing out the day sheet (record of charges and receipts). Next, Section 3 provides a simulation of jobs focusing on computerized recordkeeping. Medical Office Simulation Software (MOSS) 2.0 is included within this package as the practice management simulation software you will use to complete these activities. Section 4 includes a glossary of terms used throughout the simulation, as well as necessary forms to complete the simulation. These forms are also available for download on the Student Companion Website.

SPECIAL FEATURES

- The unique pegboard approach provides a foundational experience that helps you better understand computerized bookkeeping practices.
- The jobs include a range of experiences in accounts receivable, accounts payable, check writing, petty cash, and insurance claim form completion.
- The forms you will use are ones currently in use in physicians' offices.
- Daily and Weekly Checkups are included to ensure you are processing the information correctly.

CHANGES FROM THE FOURTH TO THE FIFTH EDITION

- All jobs in Section 2 have been updated to work in this new simulation.
- A brand-new Section 3 featuring all-new computerized case studies using practice management software, which illustrates the transition from a manual system into a computer system. This section uses the same patient case studies from the pegboard section, showing the similarities between the two systems.
- A new four-color format vividly illustrates the forms, while the reference manual's practical spiral bind makes it easy to access when you are performing tasks.
- More hands-on experience posting all types of charges and payments, managing a petty cash fund, writing checks, and keeping track of expenditures.
- Expanded information about insurance and coding concepts, including ICD-10, the latest CMS-1500 form, and a more comprehensive insurance vocabulary glossary.
- More information about the rules and regulations of HIPAA and how to protect a patient's privacy.

SUPPLEMENTS

Student Companion Website. Log on to www.cengagebrain.com and search for this book by author, title, or ISBN. Click on the link for the book to bring up the product page. Click "Access" in the Related Products & Free Materials section.

Includes the forms in Section 4 of this book, enabling you to print on demand as many copies as you need to put your skills into practice.

Instructor Companion Site. Includes an Instructor's Manual with answer keys for all jobs. Access at www.cengage.com/login with your Cengage Learning faculty account (or create a new account, following the prompts).

MOSS Information, Training, and Support Site. Access at www.cengage.com/community/moss and find information to help you use Medical Office Simulation Software (MOSS) 2.0. The site includes tutorials, frequently asked questions, documentation, and other resources to help you be successful.

ACKNOWLEDGMENTS

We would especially like to thank the many people who have provided input to make this product an excellent one. Our special thanks to:

Lorraine W. Baskin, BSc, AAS
Instructor
Heald College
Concord, CA

Mary Elizabeth W. Browder, MEd, CMA(AAMA)
Associate Professor
Raymond Walters College, University of Cincinnati
Cincinnati, OH

Billie Jean Buda, CMA
Adjunct Professor
Jackson Community College
Jackson, MI

Okezie Iroz-Nnanta, CPC
Instructor
Heald College
Milpitas, CA

Lisa Wright
Medical Assisting Program Coordinator
Bristol Community College
Fall River, MA

SECTION 1

REFERENCE MANUAL

WELCOME

You are learning to be a medical office professional. Yours is a vital and very demanding position, and the pride you have in the medical profession will help you succeed. Every day in your job you will encounter new challenges but also rewarding experiences. To help you prepare, this simulation will present typical situations that you will encounter while working in a medical front office and provide experience in both the manual and the computer systems of bookkeeping. The first part of this simulation is designed to offer hands-on practice with basic manual bookkeeping procedures. The second part of this simulation provides the experience of transferring the bookkeeping knowledge learned into a computerized system.

As a medical office professional, you are often the first person to communicate with a patient, either in person or by telephone. The medical office professional assumes a public relations role, providing a favorable first impression of your physician-employer and the medical facility. The medical office professional can offer a calm, reassuring presence when a patient is concerned about his or her own health or the health of a family member.

Confidentiality

One of the most crucial aspects of your job as a medical office professional is maintaining privacy and security of patient information. Confidentiality is not only important in patient care, it is the law. The Health Insurance Portability and Accountability Act of 1996 (HIPAA), a law administered by the U.S. Department of Health and Human Services, governs the rules and procedures providing privacy and security of a patient's health information. At the time of registration, each patient is asked to read and sign a health information release form, which is then kept on file, allowing the medical office to submit the patient's health care information to the insurance carrier for reimbursement of the patient's claim (see Figure 1-1). A notation on the submitted insurance claim states that the patient's signature is on

Douglasville Medicine Associates
5076 Brand Blvd
Douglasville, NY 01234
(123) 456-7890

Authorization to Release Health Care Information

Patient _____   Date of Birth _____

SSN _____   Previous Name _____

I request and authorize _____ to release the health care information of the patient named above to:

Name

_____

Address

_____

This request and authorization applies to: (Please initial the appropriate box)

☐ Health care information relating to the following treatment, condition, or dates of treatment:

☐ All health care information **EXCLUDING** specific information relating to sexually transmitted diseases (including HIV/AIDS), alcohol or drug use, or visits related to psychiatric disorders or mental health.

☐ All health care information **INCLUDING** specific information relating to sexually transmitted diseases (including HIV/AIDS), alcohol or drug use, or visits related to psychiatric disorders or mental health.

☐ Other:

I understand that my express consent is required to release any health care information relating to testing, diagnosis, and/or treatment of HIV (AIDS virus), sexually transmitted diseases, psychiatric disorders/mental health, or drug and/or alcohol use. If I have been tested, diagnosed, or treated for HIV (AIDS virus), sexually transmitted diseases, psychiatric disorders/mental health, or drug and/or alcohol use, you are specifically authorized to release all health care information relating to such diagnosis, testings or treatment.

_____
Signature of patient or patient's authorized representative

_____
Relationship to patient

_____
Date

AUTHORIZATION TO RELEASE MEDICAL BENEFITS

I authorize payment of medical benefits to the undersigned physician for medical services rendered.

Signed _____   Date _____

© Cengage Learning 2013

FIGURE 1-1: Authorization to Release Health Care Information.

file, thus giving permission for his or her protected health information to be released to the insurance carrier.

Each patient should be given a copy of the office's HIPAA Notice of the Privacy Practices **(see Figure 1-2)** and also sign another form acknowledging receipt of the HIPAA Notice of Privacy Practices **(see Figure 1-3)**; this form is kept in the

---

Summary of Notice of Privacy Practices

The following is a brief summary of your rights and our responsibilities as detailed in the attached **Notice of Privacy Practices (the "Notice"). This Summary is for your convenience and is not a substitute for reading the entire Notice and does not modify the terms of the Notice.**

1. **Uses and Disclosures of Your Health Information.** We may use the information we develop and collect for treatment by our practice or disclose the information to others to whom we refer you for treatment, for payment for these services, and for certain health care "operations" such as improving the competence and quality of our staff and business planning and management. We may disclose your information to our business associates, such as medical transcriptionists, billing services, and others who assist in the operations of our practice.

   We may call you to remind you of appointments and may leave a message on your answering machine if you have one. We may also disclose information to your family about your location, general condition, or death. If you are available and able, we will ask your consent first. We may also use your information to recommend products or services related to your care, but will not use or disclose your information for marketing purposes without your written authorization.

   Your medical information may be disclosed without your authorization as required by law, for public health purposes, health care oversight, including audits and investigations, judicial and administrative proceedings, subject to the limits imposed by state and federal law, and certain other purposes.

2. **Other Uses and Disclosures.** Except as described in the Notice, we will not use or disclose your medical information without your written authorization. You can revoke an authorization at any time, except to the extent that we have already taken action in reliance on the authorization.

3. **Your Health Information and Rights.** You have a number of rights under state and/or federal law, which are subject to the terms and conditions specified in the Notice:
   a. You may request restrictions on certain uses and disclosures of your information.
   b. You may request that you receive your information from us in a certain way.
   c. You may inspect and copy your medical records.
   d. You may request an amendment to any record you believe is inaccurate.
   e. You may request an accounting of disclosures made of your records.

4. **Changes to the Notice.** We reserve the right to change the Notice. If we do so, we will post it in our office, and provide a copy upon request.

5. **Complaints.** You may file a complaint to our Privacy Official whose name is above or with the federal government as detailed in the Notice. You will not be penalized for filing any complaint.

© Cengage Learning 2013

FIGURE 1-2: Notice of Privacy Practices.

Douglasville Medicine Associates
5076 Brand Blvd
Douglasville, NY 01234
(123) 456-7890

Acknowledgment of Notice of Privacy Practices

I _____, acknowledge that I have read and understood the Notice of Privacy Practices.

Signed: _____ Date: _____

© Cengage Learning 2013

FIGURE 1-3: Acknowledgment of Notice of Privacy Practices.

patient's medical record. HIPAA's Privacy Rule states that the release of information authorization remains in effect until either the expiration date listed on the form, an expiration event related to the use of the authorization form, reaching the age of majority for a minor, termination of a health plan, or the choice of the patient to rescind authorization occurs. Many offices choose to update the Authorization Release form once a year.

The medical office professional has the responsibility to keep disorders as well as the personal characteristics of patients confidential. Maintaining a patient's privacy can be accomplished by using a variety of methods, which may include:

- Discussing a patient's condition solely with your employer-physician or other personnel on a need-to-know basis.
- Conducting all confidential conversations in a private area where the conversation will not be overheard by patients or by others not involved in the patient's care.
- Being sure that telephone conversations or conversations with other medical personnel will not be overheard.
- Storing patients' files in an area accessible only to medical personnel and, if using a manual filing system, locking up medical records for privacy. If using electronic medical records (EMRs), never give out your password to co-workers.
- Storing all sensitive material out of sight of others coming to the reception desk.
- Keeping the computer screen facing away from others approaching the reception desk; using the locking mechanism on the computer when away from the desk; never sharing computer passwords with others; and changing passwords frequently to ensure privacy.
- Posting the physician's daily list in a location unnoticed by patients because it specifies the nature of a patient's illness.
- Always obtaining written authorization by patients or by parents of minor patients before releasing any medical records. (This is often handled through a release statement signed by the patient on his or her first visit to the medical office; recall the form shown in Figure 1-1.)

Breaches of confidentiality could embarrass patients or even lead to a malpractice suit. Extend this respect for privacy to your experiences with other workers and to any knowledge you may have about your physician-employer's personal life. When newly hired, you may be asked to sign an Employee Confidentiality Statement (**see Figure 1-4**).

Documentation

Another crucial aspect of the medical professional's role is documenting procedures, messages, and other pertinent patient information. Documentation, whether it is in a message or a medical record, needs to be complete, correct, legible, and professional. Documentation should be done preferably using permanent black ink, although blue ink is acceptable in many facilities; the rationale being that documentation in black tends to photocopy better than inks of other colors. Facilities or hospitals that are open for different shifts often use a different color ink for each shift. Pencils or erasable ink should not be used for documentation, because they will not provide a permanent record of the documentation. Correction fluid (such as

---

Douglasville Medicine Associates
5076 Brand Blvd
Douglasville, NY 01234
(123) 456-7890

Employee Confidentiality Statement

As an employee of _____ (employer), and having been trained as an administrative medical assistant with employee responsibilities and authorization to access personal medical and health information, I recognize that violation of confidentiality statutes and rules may lead to immediate dismissal from employment and, depending on state laws, criminal prosecution. I understand that such violation may cause irreparable damage to my employer, and the employer and any other injured party may seek legal action against me. I acknowledge that this signed document will be placed in my personnel file at this facility.

_____   _____
Signature   Witness signature

_____
Print Name

_____
Date

© Cengage Learning 2013

FIGURE 1-4: Employee Confidentiality Statement.

Wite-Out®) should not be used, nor should any content be erased or scribbled, removing or obscuring the content entered in error. Medical records are considered legal documents and, although necessary for quality patient care, the documentation may be used in court should the need arise. All entries made by the medical office professional should be signed using a legal name and credentials. Procedures and communications that are not documented in the medical record are legally considered not done. The proper method to correct an error made in a medical document is to, carefully draw a single line through the error (usually in red ink), write "correction" above the error, make the correction, and date and initial the correction (**see Figure 1-5**). An error made in an EMR can be corrected immediately if noticed, or an error noted at a later date would be corrected following the procedure in the operator's manual of the computer system being used.

4:30 EF 3/4/2013
3/4/2013 2:30 p.m. BP 186/92 E.Flores, MA—

© Cengage Learning 2013

FIGURE 1-5: Correcting an Error in a Paper Medical Record.

Always remember that your first priority is patient care. That involves knowing your scope of practice. You are a trained medical professional, but you are not a physician; therefore, you do not give medical advice or diagnose a patient's condition. Direct all detailed questions regarding patient treatment to your physician-employer.

PROCEDURE 1: COMMUNICATIONS IN A MEDICAL FACILITY

In this simulation, you are employed at the Douglasville Medicine Associates, a family practice, located at 5076 Brand Blvd, Suite 401, in Douglasville, New York. You will be working with Dr. L. D. Heath, a board-certified physician in family practice. The office hours are Monday through Friday, 9:00 a.m. to 5:00 p.m. During the lunch hour, noon to 1:00 p.m., all incoming calls are automatically routed to an answering service.

As a medical office professional, you work from 8:00 a.m. to 5:00 p.m., Monday through Friday. The office staff includes another full-time medical professional and two part-time employees.

This simulation will describe the typical duties and activities of a medical office professional working at Douglasville Medicine Associates during one workweek. You will be provided with all necessary background to complete this simulation first manually and then by computer. The activities to be completed by you in this simulation are marked as jobs.

All forms needed for this simulation are provided in Section 4 of this book or within the package. Alternately, you may download additional forms from the Student Companion Website. Before beginning each job, make sure you have located all the correct forms.

Telephone Voice

The telephone is an important piece of equipment in a medical office. The first contact a patient may have with a medical office is by telephone and it is essential that the medical professional has good telephone techniques. Something as simple as the way the telephone is answered can have an effect on the patient's impression of the medical office and the care they may receive. When answering the telephone, begin by saying, "Douglasville Medicine Associates, [your name] speaking. How may I help you?"

Smile while you are talking on the telephone. It is hard to be unpleasant when you are smiling, and your cheerful appearance will demonstrate enthusiasm to those around you. Remember to speak clearly, calmly, not too fast, and at a moderate volume. The tone of the medical professional's voice should convey warmth and friendliness since the first contact with a caller is important in making a good impression. Even if a patient becomes angry or offensive, the medical professional should remain poised, in control, and nonargumentative. One of the responsibilities of the medical office professional is to screen or **triage** calls, meaning to prioritize the urgency of the call. Specific questions, which often are found in the office's procedure manual or triage manual, must be asked to gather pertinent information from the patient that will be used to make an appropriate judgment of the urgency of the call (**see Figure 1-6**). Being able to recognize an emergency situation or when it is necessary to schedule a patient for an urgent visit is important in providing the best care to patients.

- What happened?
- Is the patient breathing?
- Is the patient bleeding? How much? From where?
- Is the patient conscious?
- Does the patient have an elevated temperature? If yes, what is it?
- Did the patient ingest something toxic? What was it? How much? How long ago? Do you have the container?

© Cengage Learning 2013

FIGURE 1-6: Screening Questions to Ask When Assessing the Urgency of a Call.

The physicians at Douglasville Medicine Associates have assigned the following priority to incoming telephone calls and listed them in the office policy manual as:

1. Calls that must go through to a physician immediately
2. Calls for which the physician must be interrupted immediately for instructions
3. Calls to be returned by the physician between patients
4. Calls to be returned at the convenience of the physician
5. Calls that require instructions from the physician; the medical office professional calls back to convey the information (such as prescription refills)
6. Calls for appointments, cancellations, and rescheduling appointments
7. Calls from patients requesting information regarding the status of their accounts

See **Figure 1-7** for how to handle incoming calls to the medical office.

Calls Handled by the Front Office Professional	Calls Handled by the Physician
1. New and established appointments	1. Emergency calls from hospital and patients
2. Questions regarding billing and insurance	2. Abnormal laboratory results
3. Prescription refill information	3. Other physicians
4. Favorable laboratory reports	4. Medical questions from patients and their families
5. General information about the medical facility	

© Cengage Learning 2013

FIGURE 1-7: Handling Incoming Calls in a Medical Office.

Recording Messages

Taking or recording accurate messages can be accomplished by using a telephone pad that may be purchased at any office supply store. Specific information needs to be obtained from the caller in order for a complete record of the call and a satisfactory action to occur. The minimal information that should be obtained includes:

- Caller's full, legal name; many offices request date of birth (DOB) and insurance information
- Telephone number: where the caller can be reached during the day or after hours (i.e., cell phone number, home number, work number)
- Who the call is for (i.e., a specific physician, billing department, office nurse)
- Reason for the call (i.e., prescription refill, request for a written note, question about bill)
- Urgency of the call (i.e., routine questions about medical practice, sudden illness needing immediate attention)
- Action to be taken (i.e., return call by physician or other office personnel, written note as requested by patient)
- Name or initials of the person taking the call

After completing a message, the medical office professional should read back the information to the caller to be sure of the accuracy of the message.

If the caller is requesting a call-back from the physician or the office for a non-emergency reason, it is always a good policy to give the caller an approximate time when the call might be made according to the policies of the office. For example, many offices make return calls after office hours so that the physician will have uninterrupted time to talk with the patient. A simple statement such as, "The doctor usually returns calls at the end of the workday, which would be after 5 p.m. today," is helpful; this way the patient is not sitting around by the telephone waiting for the call.

Placing a Caller on Hold

A caller should never be put on hold until the medical office professional knows who is calling and why, so that an emergency situation will not be missed. Before any call is put on hold, the medical office professional should ask for and receive permission from the caller. Once permission is given for the caller to be put on hold, the caller should not be left unattended for more than 30 to 40 seconds. If the call cannot go through within that time, the caller should be given the option of continuing to hold or the option of a return call. The medical office professional can take down the caller's number and a short message (documenting the information discussed in the previous section) and have the call returned when the line is free.

Transferring a Call

With multiple telephone lines in a busy medical office, the medical office professional may need to transfer a call directly to the person who may best be able to help the caller. When answering an incoming call needing to be transferred to another extension, the medical office professional should ask for the caller's name, telephone number, and a short description of the reason for the call. This information will allow the call to be directed to the appropriate person or department while providing insight as to the reason for the call if needed. The caller's name and telephone number may also be used to redial the caller should the line become disconnected. Many offices provide the caller with the telephone number and extension of the individual he or she is trying to reach, allowing the caller to make a direct call if the person is not available or a message is not left.

Outgoing Telephone Calls

Outgoing calls should be made in a private area where the conversation will not be overheard, especially if the material to be communicated is of a sensitive or private nature. Care should be taken to speak only to the person for whom the call is intended, and if a patient approves that a message may be left on the answering machine, only a general message of "please call the office" should be left.

Fax Machines

A convenient, easy-to-use piece of equipment in a medical facility is the fax machine. Patient reports, prescription information from pharmacies, test results, and consent forms are just a few examples of the types of documents that can be sent or received via fax machines. The advantages of using a fax machine instead of the U.S. mail are speed and convenience; the disadvantage is confidentiality. Not all fax machines are located in a secure area where the message is sent to the person for whom it was intended. The fax can be sent to a mailroom where any passerby can read the contents of the fax. Security issues can be managed by following a few simple rules such as:

- Calling ahead to be sure the appropriate person will be available to receive the fax.
- Attaching a cover letter indicating that the material being sent is of a sensitive or confidential nature and that it is against state and federal laws to disclose the contents of the fax. Material that is extremely confidential should not be sent by fax if at all possible.
- Extreme care should be taken to dial the correct number, placing a call to verify that the fax was received, and printing a receipt copy for the message, which is then kept in the patient's medical record.

Encryption, a technology that converts information into codes, can be used to provide and protect confidentiality of information sent. However, encryption requires the cooperation of both the sender and the receiver in order to be used.

E-mails

E-mail sends messages over computer lines, in contrast to faxes, which use telephone lines, although both are convenient methods of sending messages. Many offices use e-mail to send reminders to patients about appointments rather than making telephone calls. Patients can send messages to the medical office such as a cancellation of an appointment and when printed out can be placed in the patient's medical record for documentation of the cancelled appointment. E-mails are also a convenient way to send notices to all departments in an office or to create a calendar of events and meetings.

All e-mails should be written in a professional manner and should avoid time-sensitive material that might be overlooked, causing someone to miss an urgent or important meeting if the e-mail was not read in a timely manner.

Incoming Mail

Another responsibility of the front office professional is to handle incoming mail. All incoming mail, including faxes, certified or registered letters, personal letters, letters from insurance companies, advertising, periodicals, catalogs, and pharmaceutical supplies, should be sorted according to category in order to speed up delivery to the appropriate department or person prior to opening. Dr. Heath has requested that the mail be classified and sorted as follows:

1. Registered, certified letters, and other important mail for consideration
2. Patient laboratory and test results
   a. Negative results should be attached to the patient's medical record and placed on the physician's desk for immediate attention.
3. Payments
   a. Checks from insurance companies
   b. Checks from patients
4. Medical and other health-related journals
5. Magazines for the reception area
6. Throwaway items such as circulars and advertisements
7. Do not open mail marked "personal" or "confidential." Place this mail unopened on the physician's desk.

Once the mail is sorted and delivered to the appropriate person or department, you may open and handle the contents of the envelopes as directed by office policies or referred to the appropriate person or department, depending on the size and personnel of the facility. Remember that any paper item containing a patient's name or containing private information needs to be shredded before discarded.

PROCEDURE 2: SCHEDULING

You will maintain a weekly calendar for Dr. Heath for the week of March 4–8 (**see Figure 1-8**). You will record personal and professional appointments entered in the weekly calendar in Dr. Heath's appointment book as well. The calendar acts as a reminder to Dr. Heath and allows the office staff to reach him in an emergency.

| | | | March — | | | |
Sunday	Monday	Tuesday	Wednesday	Thursday	Friday	Saturday
					1	**2**
3	**4** 3-5 p.m. Hospital rounds 5 p.m. Family practice dinner meeting	**5** 9-10 a.m. Staff breakfast at hospital 4 p.m. Lecture at Douglasville CC	**6** 12-1 p.m. Lunch seminar at the hospital	**7** 5 p.m. Hospital staff meeting	**8**	**9**

FIGURE 1-8: Weekly Calendar for Dr. Heath.

Appointment Book Matrix

After selecting an appointment book that has suitable space for the number of physicians, the time slots, and hours available for the type of medical practice, the **matrix** needs to be set up. Setting up the matrix is the process of accurately marking off the times and days that the office or physician will not be available for appointments, such as meetings, hospital rounds, days the office will be closed, or vacation days. The times for patient appointments will be clearly visible and prevent errors in scheduling. The matrix needs to be set up before appointments can be entered, regardless of whether the medical practice uses a manual or a computer appointment scheduling system. Many offices tend to leave available slots in the schedule to allow for appointments for patients needing same day care; these are sometimes called "Emergency Slots." In a manual system, pencil should be used because the matrix can change, and, if done in ink, it will be difficult to amend and become illegible. A hard copy of the schedule should be made for legal purposes.

A computerized system also has the ability to create hard copies of the schedule for legal purposes, should the need arise.

Scheduling Styles

There are many different types of scheduling styles that may be used in a medical facility. Each office selects the type of scheduling style, or combination of scheduling styles, that best suits the type of medical practice. The types of scheduling styles include:

- *Open hours:* No appointments are necessary and patients are seen on a first-come basis throughout the hours the facility is open. However, emergencies take preference over any patient waiting in the reception area.

Although convenient, some patients may end up waiting a long time before they are seen by the physician.

- *Wave:* Three patients are scheduled for each hour and seen in the order that they arrived. For example, if three patients are scheduled for 1:00 p.m., estimating that if each patient takes 20 minutes, three patients will be seen in an hour. Because not all patients take the same amount of time, if patient 1 finishes up a bit early, patient 2 is already in the office and is able to go in for the appointment. If patient 2 goes past the 20 minutes allowed, patient 3 should be seen on time because patient 2 went in earlier. The goal is to complete three patients each hour.

- *Modified wave:* Two patients are scheduled at the top of the hour and one patient at half past the hour. The goal is the same as the wave style of scheduling, three patients per hour, but with the hope of eliminating the 40-minute wait to see the physician for the last person to arrive.

- *Clustering:* A scheduling style similar to a production-line setup, and sometimes called "grouping," is the process of scheduling patients having similar procedures or having similar problems grouped together to increase efficiency. This type of scheduling style is commonly used in offices for flu shot clinics, well-baby check-ups, school physicals, or routine pregnancy visits. Patients are booked consecutively and blocks of time are recorded in the appointment book.

- *Double-booking:* Booking two patients to see the physician at the same time is not recommended because a backup of patients can occur if all patients show up. Double-booking can be useful in a medical practice if the patients need to see other health care providers as well as the physician during the visit. For example, the patient coming for a complete physical exam (CP) may go to one department for blood work, then have an electrocardiogram (**EKG**) done in another section of the facility before going in to see the physician. If two or three patients were scheduled for the same time, each patient would go to a separate department and rotate so no patient would be sitting and waiting for a long time before receiving care.

- *Stream:* One of the most common styles of scheduling used in medical facilities consists of a separate appointment time for each patient throughout the workday, the time allowed depending on the reason for the visit. Each office sets up the amount of time given to each patient depending on the physical facilities available (number of exam rooms), the type of medical practice (surgical procedures may take longer than medical procedures), and the work habits and preferences of the physicians (some physicians like to work at a faster pace than others).

- *Practice-based:* A combination of scheduling styles is usually referred to as "practiced-based." For example, a physician's office may use clustering one or two mornings a week and stream scheduling the rest of the time.

You are responsible for scheduling appointments during the set office hours. The appointment intervals have been set and approved by the physicians of Douglasville Medicine Associates. Normally, in this practice, appointments for established patients are scheduled every 15 minutes for office visits that meet the specifications listed by the **Current Procedural Terminology (CPT) codes**. If a diagnostic procedure (such as an EKG) is to be performed, however, the patient may be scheduled for a 30-minute visit. New patient physical examinations, as well as other diagnostic or treatment procedures are scheduled as 45- to 60-minute visits. A portion of each day is set aside for emergencies; no regular appointments are scheduled during these times. Although various styles of scheduling may be used in a medical practice, the most important aspect of scheduling is flexibility, as well as sensitivity for meeting the needs of the patient.

Scheduling Information

Patients arrange for new and return appointments either in person (before they leave the office) or by telephone. Be sure to obtain the following information when scheduling an appointment for either an established patient or a new patient:

- *Patient's name and date of birth (DOB).* Be sure you obtain the correct spelling of both the first and the last name. Many offices require the patient's date of birth (DOB) as a second patient identifier to ensure scheduling the correct patient, because patients can have the same name. Computerized scheduling systems may require DOB when scheduling a patient.

- *Nature of illness.* The nature of the illness or the type of examination will determine the amount of time you schedule for each appointment. Involved details are not necessary but enough information needs to be collected in order to assess the urgency of the appointment and to provide the patient with enough time to receive quality care.

- *Telephone number.* Obtain a daytime telephone number, such as a cell phone number, in case you need to contact a patient during office hours for additional information or to reschedule an appointment.

- *Insurance or payment information.* Obtain these data for new patients when an appointment is made to be sure the physician is participating in the patient's insurance (this is discussed further in the insurance section). Although this information is already on file for established patients, it is a good idea to ask about any changes in insurance because an insurance change may affect reimbursement. If a computerized scheduling system is used, the type of insurance and the insurance number is usually required.

Figure 1-9 shows a completed appointment book page for March 4 in Dr. Heath's appointment book. Figure 1-9 will provide you with information you will need for the simulation.

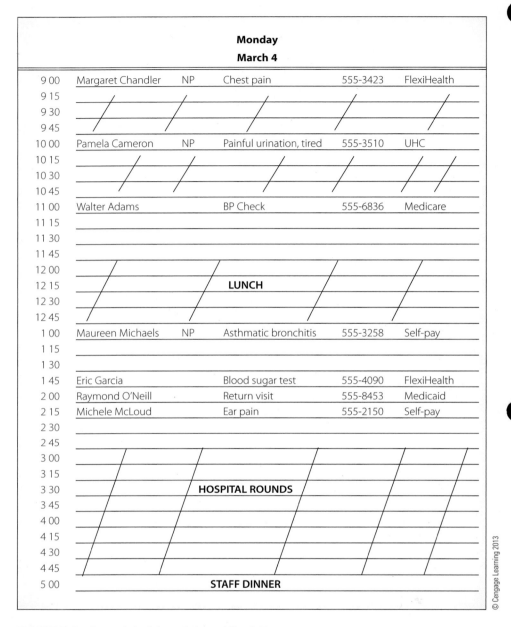

FIGURE 1-9: Completed Appointment Book Page.

HIV positive is one of many sensitive diagnoses and confidentiality should be maintained. A sensitive diagnosis should not be entered in the appointment book. If a patient's appointment was for the results of a HIV test, a notation of "lab work results" would be sufficient information to enter into the appointment schedule rather than "HIV lab results." If more information is needed by the medical office professional, it can usually be obtained in the medical record or by asking the physician.

PROCEDURE 3: PATIENT LIST AND DAILY APPOINTMENT WORKSHEET

At the end of each day, you will prepare the following day's Patient List. The manual appointment book is written in pencil and therefore cannot be considered a legal document; however, a computer printout is considered a legal document. The manual appointment book can be photocopied to produce a legal record of patient visits or the patient list may be used to provide a permanent hard copy of the patients scheduled for the day and the reason for the scheduled visits. The Patient List provides the physician with necessary information about the patients that will be examined each day as well as provide a legal copy of the patients being cared for each day. In the event the computer system fails, the list can be helpful in identifying the patients scheduled for the day. The list can also be used by the medical office professional to pull patient medical records to place on the physician's desk.

Some offices may prepare a Daily Appointment Worksheet instead of a Patient List. A Daily Appointment Worksheet differs from the Patient List because it lists not only the patients and the reason for the visits scheduled but all the other scheduled activities of the day such as lunch times and meetings. The Daily Appointment Worksheet can be photocopied from the appointment book in the manual system or generated on the computer system by a printout. It is up to the discretion of the medical facility whether to use a Patient List or a Daily Appointment Worksheet; in this simulation, a Patient List is used.

Because the "Nature of Illness" should be confidential, placement of the Patient List should be done with discretion, keeping it out of view of nonmedical personnel. The data you need to prepare the Patient List is available from the appointment book. The Patient List contains the following information:

- Day and date
- Time each patient is to be seen and the length of time scheduled
- Name of the patient
- Procedure to be performed
- Nature of the illness, if applicable

Figure 1-10 shows the Patient List for Monday, March 4, and also provides information needed for the simulation.

PROCEDURE 4: PATIENT REGISTRATION SHEET

When a new patient arrives for a scheduled appointment, he or she is asked to complete a patient registration form **(see Figure 1-11)** that shows typical information requested, although each office uses its own format. The completed patient registration form provides the data needed to prepare a patient ledger card in a manual system **(see Figure 1-12)** or input into a computer system. (Data for completing a ledger card or computer record for a hospitalized new patient will be provided by your physician-employer from hospital records.) A new patient is also asked to complete a Health History form **(see Figure 1-13)**, which will provide the physician with valuable information about the patient's past and present health issues.

		Patient List		
		Monday		
		March 4		

Hour	Patient	Procedure	Nature of Illness	Time
9 00	Margaret Chandler	NP	Chest pain	60 min
~~9 15~~				
~~9 30~~				
~~9 45~~				
10 00	Pamela Cameron	NP	Painful urination, tired	60 min
~~10 15~~				
~~10 30~~				
~~10 45~~				
11 00	Walter Adams	Return visit	BP Check	15 min
11 15				
11 30				
11 45				
~~12 00~~				
~~12 15~~				
~~12 30~~				
~~12 45~~				
1 00	Maureen Michaels	NP	Asthmatic bronchitis	45 min
~~1 15~~				
~~1 30~~				
1 45	Eric Garcia	Return visit	Blood sugar test	15 min
2 00	Raymond O'Neill	Return visit		15 min
2 15	Michelle McLoud	Return visit	Ear pain	15 min
2 30				
2 45				
~~3 00~~				
~~3 15~~				
~~3 30~~				
~~3 45~~				
~~4 00~~				
~~4 15~~				
~~4 30~~				
~~4 45~~				
~~5 00~~				

FIGURE 1-10: Daily Appointment Worksheet.

Authorization Forms

Authorization to release health care information is another essential form signed by new patients or according to the policy of the medical office. Some offices require new authorization forms each year and many require a new form to be signed if the patient's insurance carrier has changed (refer back to Figure 1-1).

PATIENT INFORMATION   Date _____

Name _____ Sex _____

Street address _____

City _____ State _____ Zip Code _____

Phone number _____ (home) _____ (work)

Birth date _____ Social Security Number _____

For minor patient: Name/address of responsible party (identify relationship)

_____

For adult: Name and address of spouse/nearest relative (identify relationship)

_____

Patient's employer information _____

_____

Name and address of primary insurance carrier (list others on back of sheet)

_____

Group number _____ Identification number _____

Name and date of birth of policyholder _____

Employer of policyholder (if different from patient) _____

_____

Referred by _____

Any known allergies? _____

_____

Past medical history _____

_____

_____

I hereby authorize information to be furnished to insurance carriers and/or attorneys concerning my illness and treatments and I hereby assign the physician all payments for medical services rendered to me or my dependents. I certify that all information provided above is true and accurate to the best of my knowledge.

Date _____ Signature _____

FIGURE 1-11: Patient Information Form.

PROCEDURE 5: BOOKKEEPING SYSTEMS

Many types of bookkeeping systems may be used in medical offices and they range from simple to complex. Many offices are becoming computerized, but a basic knowledge of the bookkeeping and accounting functions is essential in managing the finances of a medical office.

STATEMENT

L.D. Heath, M.D.
Douglasville Medicine Associates
5076 Brand Blvd, Ste 401
Douglasville, NY 01234
(123) 456-7890

Ms. Helen J. Baldwin
1975 Van Dyke Road
Douglasville, NY 01234

DATE	REFERENCE	DESCRIPTION	CHARGES		CREDITS PYMNTS.		ADJ.		BALANCE	
			BALANCED FORWARD							
3/4	Helen	99213	80	00	10	00	—	—	70	00

RB40BC-2-96   PLEASE PAY LAST AMOUNT IN BALANCE COLUMN ⬆

THIS IS A COPY OF YOUR ACCOUNT AS IT APPEARS ON OUR RECORDS

TELEPHONE	SPOUSE NAME	DATE OF BIRTH	SOC. SEC. NO	DRIVERS LIC. NO.
(123)555-0086	Kenneth	11/13/1946	407-52-7430	

EMPLOYER: CITY - STATE - PHONE	SPOUSE EMPLOYER: CITY - STATE - PHONE
Retired	Temporary Employment Center
	1400 Parkside Ave
	Douglasville, NY 01234 (123)555-2266

NAME-ADDRESS-PHONE OF NEAREST RELATIVE	OTHERS PROF. SERVICE USED: CITY - STATE - PHONE
Kenneth (spouse)	
DOB: 1/30/1946	
SOC, Sec. No: 024-66-1052	

CREDIT/INSURANCE INFORMATION
Commercial Company Insurance ID#293153J (Kenneth)

OWN ☐   RENT ☐

COMMENTS
Signature on file, accepts assignment
HIPAA form: signed and given to pt

USE LEAD PENCIL- FELT TIP MARKER-TYPEWRITER

FIGURE 1-12: Completed Ledger Card, Front and Back.

Manual System

In this simulation, as a medical office professional employed by family practice physicians, you will handle typical record-keeping activities. To record these activities, you will first use a pegboard (write-it-once) system and then a computerized system. The first part of the simulation gives the user hands-on experience with a pegboard system to offer a clear understanding of the bookkeeping processes of entering charges and payments. It is usually easier to begin with a pegboard system because it demonstrates everyday accounting principles and the handling of a patient's account from start to finish. This knowledge can then be easily adapted to a computer system. A pegboard system consists of ledger cards, day sheets, receipts, and superbills.

Computerized System

The second part of this simulation demonstrates how to enter the information gathered in the pegboard system into a computerized system. Basically, the same information is being entered but in a different manner. Because a computer system can shut down unexpectedly, it is beneficial for the medical office professional to understand the pegboard bookkeeping process in order to maintain accurate patient accounts without the aid of the computer.

PROCEDURE 6: THE PEGBOARD SYSTEM

The pegboard system is a commonly used write-it-once system of record-keeping. Certain data, such as the name of the patient, fees charged, payments, adjustments, and balance due, are recorded in such a way that they appear on multiple records using some forms with a carbon strip and other non-carbon-required (NCR) forms. The specially treated forms used in this system eliminate the necessity and cost associated with manually rewriting data. The pegboard is a flat writing surface with a series of pegs positioned along the left edge. Special forms are properly aligned on top of each other on the pegboard. When the system is used properly, all data recorded with a ballpoint pen on the top form is simultaneously reproduced on each form lying beneath it. The pegboard system is an effective way to record accounts receivable, accounts payable, and payroll, because several records containing identical data may be prepared in one writing. The chance of introducing error as numbers are copied by hand from one record to another is lessened. Medical offices can benefit from the economy and accuracy of the pegboard system without having to buy expensive machines or use specially trained operators. Some offices use the pegboard system as a backup to their computer system or to keep track of co-payments received from patients.

Ledger Cards

Ledger cards are used to provide a permanent record of data on each patient and the status of his or her account. Many offices photocopy the front side of the ledger

HEALTH HISTORY
(Confidential)

Name _____ Today's date _____

Age _____ Birthdate _____ Date of last physical examination _____

What is your reason for visit? _____

MEDICATIONS: List medications you are currently taking.	ALLERGIES: To medications or substances

Pharmacy name _____ Phone _____

SYMPTOMS: Check (✔) symptoms you currently have or have had in the past.

GENERAL	GASTROINTESTINAL	EYE, EAR, NOSE, THROAT	MEN only
☐ Chills	☐ Appetite poor	☐ Bleeding gums	☐ Breast lump
☐ Depression	☐ Bloating	☐ Blurred vision	☐ Erection difficulties
☐ Dizziness	☐ Bowel changes	☐ Crossed eyes	☐ Lump in testicles
☐ Fainting	☐ Constipation	☐ Difficulty swallowing	☐ Penis discharge
☐ Fever	☐ Diarrhea	☐ Double vision	☐ Sore on penis
☐ Forgetfulness	☐ Excessive hunger	☐ Earache	☐ Other
☐ Headache	☐ Excessive thirst	☐ Ear discharge	
☐ Loss of sleep	☐ Gas	☐ Hay fever	**WOMEN only**
☐ Loss of weight	☐ Hemorrhoids	☐ Hoarseness	☐ Abnormal Pap smear
☐ Nervousness	☐ Indigestion	☐ Loss of hearing	☐ Bleeding between periods
☐ Numbness	☐ Nausea	☐ Nosebleeds	☐ Breast lump
☐ Sweats	☐ Rectal bleeding	☐ Persistent cough	☐ Extreme menstrual pain
	☐ Stomach pain	☐ Ringing in ears	☐ Hot flashes
MUSCLE/JOINT/BONE	☐ Vomiting	☐ Sinus problems	☐ Nipple discharge
Pain, weakness, numbness in:	☐ Vomiting blood	☐ Vision — Flashes	☐ Painful intercourse
☐ Arms ☐ Hips		☐ Vision — Halos	☐ Vaginal discharge
☐ Back ☐ Legs	**CARDIOVASCULAR**		☐ Other
☐ Feet ☐ Neck	☐ Chest pain	**SKIN**	Date of last
☐ Hands ☐ Shoulders	☐ High blood pressure	☐ Bruise easily	menstrual period _____
	☐ Irregular heart beat	☐ Hives	Date of last
GENITO-URINARY	☐ Low blood pressure	☐ Itching	Pap smear _____
☐ Blood in urine	☐ Poor circulation	☐ Change in moles	Have you had
☐ Frequent urination	☐ Rapid heart beat	☐ Rash	a mammogram? _____
☐ Lack of bladder control	☐ Swelling of ankles	☐ Scars	Are you pregnant? _____
☐ Painful urination	☐ Varicose veins	☐ Sore that won't heal	Number of children _____

CONDITIONS: Check (✔) conditions you have or have had in the past.

☐ AIDS	☐ Chemical dependency	☐ High cholesterol	☐ Prostate problem
☐ Alcoholism	☐ Chicken pox	☐ HIV positive	☐ Psychiatric care
☐ Anemia	☐ Diabetes	☐ Kidney disease	☐ Rheumatic fever
☐ Anorexia	☐ Emphysema	☐ Liver disease	☐ Scarlet fever
☐ Appendicitis	☐ Epilepsy	☐ Measles	☐ Stroke
☐ Arthritis	☐ Glaucoma	☐ Migraine headaches	☐ Suicide attempt
☐ Asthma	☐ Goiter	☐ Miscarriage	☐ Thyroid problem
☐ Bleeding disorders	☐ Gonorrhea	☐ Mononucleosis	☐ Tonsillitis
☐ Breast lump	☐ Gout	☐ Multiple sclerosis	☐ Tuberculosis
☐ Bronchitis	☐ Heart disease	☐ Mumps	☐ Typhoid fever
☐ Bulimia	☐ Hepatitis	☐ Pacemaker	☐ Ulcers
☐ Cancer	☐ Hernia	☐ Pneumonia	☐ Vaginal infections
☐ Cataracts	☐ Herpes	☐ Polio	☐ Venereal disease

FIGURE 1-13: Patient Health History Form.

(All information is strictly confidential)

FAMILY HISTORY: Fill in health information about your family.

Relation	Age	State of Health	Age at Death	Cause of Death	Check (✓) if your blood relatives had any of the following: Disease	Relationship to you
					Arthritis, gout	
					Asthma, hay fever	
					Cancer	
					Chemical dependency	
					Diabetes	
					Hear disease, strokes	
					High blood pressure	
					Kidney disease	
					Tuberculosis	
					Other	

HOSPITALIZATIONS

Year	Hospital	Reason for Hospitalization and Outcome

PREGNANCY HISTORY

Year of Birth	Sex of Birth	Complications if any

HEALTH HABITS: Check (✓) which substances you use and describe how much you use.

Caffeine	
Tobacco	
Drugs	
Other	

Have you ever had a blood transfusion? ☐ Yes ☐ No

If yes, please give approximate dates: _____

SERIOUS ILLNESS/INJURIES

SERIOUS ILLNESS/INJURIES	DATE	OUTCOME

OCCUPATIONAL CONCERNS: Check (✓) if your work exposes you to the following:

Stress	
Hazardous substances	
Heavy lifting	
Other	
Your occupation:	

I certify that the above information is correct to the best of my knowledge. I will not hold my doctor or any members of his/her staff responsible for any errors or omissions that I may have made in the completion of this form.

_____   _____
Signature   Date

_____   _____
Reviewed by   Date

FIGURE 1-13: (continued)

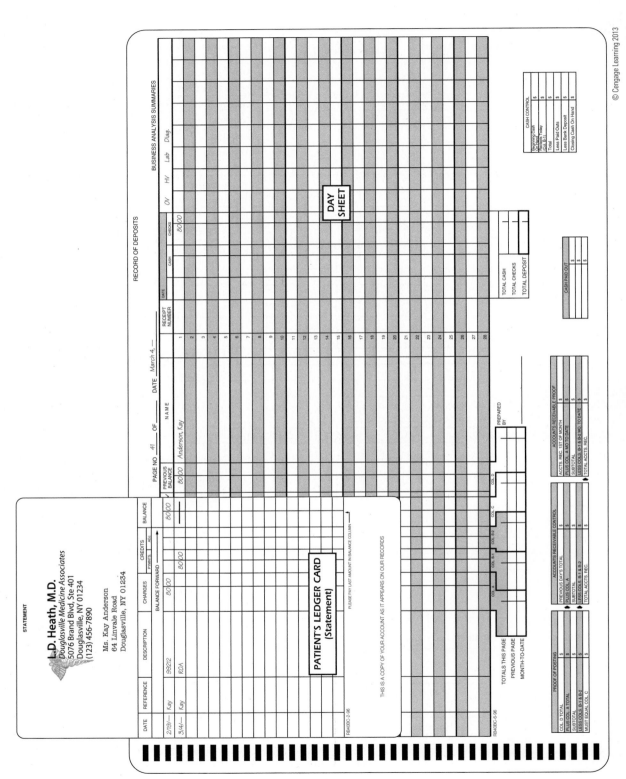

FIGURE 1-14: Pegboard System Set Up to Record Charges and Payments.

© Cengage Learning 2013

card and mail the copy to the patient as an account statement, or bill. The word *statement,* therefore, appears at the top of the ledger card. The reverse side of the ledger card includes an area in which to enter personal information about the patient such as telephone numbers, name of a spouse or an emergency contact person, Social Security number, insurance information, and a space to indicate that the patient's signature which is needed to release information to the insurance carrier is on file. This is the same information that would be entered about the patient in a computerized system. Refer back to Figure 1-12 for a completed ledger card (front and back).

Day Sheet

The day sheet is the part of the pegboard system used to record daily patient transactions such as charges and payments, record of cash and checks for deposit, a cash control table for petty cash expenditures, and current up-to-date information on bookkeeping data for the day and month. Although day sheets may vary, most collect and process similar information. Each new workday, the previous day's sheet is removed and a new day sheet is placed on the pegboard and numbered consecutively. The information from the previous day is entered on the new day sheet in specified areas. Because the day sheets have NCR forms, each sheet must be removed or the information recorded on the top sheet will be transferred to the day sheet below and may obscure the entries.

Receipts and Superbills

A receipt is usually given to a patient who makes a payment on a previously owed account and usually records the date, the patient's name, a brief description of the services provided, the charge, adjustment, payment, a balance (if any), and the date and time of the next appointment. A superbill (also known as an encounter form or charge slip) is a more detailed form listing more than just the name and address information of the physician's office. In this simulation, this form will be referred to as a superbill. The superbill is a three-part form that may be used for reimbursement from an insurance carrier if a patient is to submit his or her own insurance claim because it itemizes the services provided listing the Current Procedural Terminology (CPT) procedure codes, the ICD-CM *(International Classification of Diseases, Clinical Modification)* diagnosis codes needed by the insurance carrier to process a claim, the charges, and the balance due. Superbills may be customized for the office, and many have a space available to include the date and time of the next appointment. In this simulation, you will complete a superbill only for specified patients or for those patients who request this form, and other patients will receive receipts, although in many offices superbills are given to all patients. By the end of this simulation you will have experience with both receipts and superbills.

PROCEDURE 7: RECORDING ENTRIES IN THE PEGBOARD SYSTEM

In a typical pegboard system, the day sheet, patient's ledger card, and receipt or superbill are aligned so that each overlaps another. The specially ordered forms have holes punched in the left side so that the forms may be held in place by the pegs on the board. When you enter information along the top of a receipt or superbill, it is simultaneously recorded on the proper line of the patient's ledger card through a carbon strip that runs across the back of the receipt or superbill. The same information is also recorded on the day sheet, since the back of the ledger card and the front of the day sheet are chemically coated with an NCR substance. When the two surfaces come into contact with each other and pressure is applied, information recorded on the front of the ledger card is reproduced on the day sheet. Additional information, such as special diagnosis codes or the date of the next appointment, may be added later to individual forms. Each new workday, a new day sheet is placed on the pegboard, making sure that the top hole of the sheet is placed over the top peg of the board. The date and page number are written at the top of each page, starting with the first day of each year that the office is open. For example, March 4, page 43 will be used for the first day of this simulation.

The Business Analysis Summaries columns, which are on the far right of the day sheet, are labeled from left to right. In this simulation, place the labels Office Visits, Hospital Visits, Laboratory, and Diagnostic in the columns. Each medical facility may label the columns in the business analysis summaries columns according to the needs of its facility. For the system to work properly, the forms must be properly aligned.

Posting Charges and Payments Using a Receipt

To record payments requiring a receipt, you will need to record information simultaneously on the receipt, the ledger card, and the day sheet. A patient ledger card from the files for an established patient or a prepared ledger card for a new patient is placed under the top shingle of the receipt forms. Receipt forms come in a group, or shingle, attached together for easier attachment to the pegboard. Place a shingle of receipts over the pegs so that the carbon strip of the top receipt is aligned with the first open writing line of the day sheet. Be sure to continue the numbering consecutively when adding a new shingle of receipts to the pegboard. Place the patient's ledger card under the top receipt so that the first open writing line of the card is aligned with the carbon strip. Be sure that the columns of the patient's ledger card align exactly with the columns on the day sheet and receipt (see **Figure 1-15**). Complete the receipt as follows:

1. Enter the date in the date column.
2. Enter the patient's first name in the reference column. Many offices using a pegboard system have one ledger card per family and the patient's first name is entered in the reference column to identify which member of the family received care.
3. Enter the CPT code in the description column. The CPT codes and charges are found on the inside cover of the textbook for easy access.

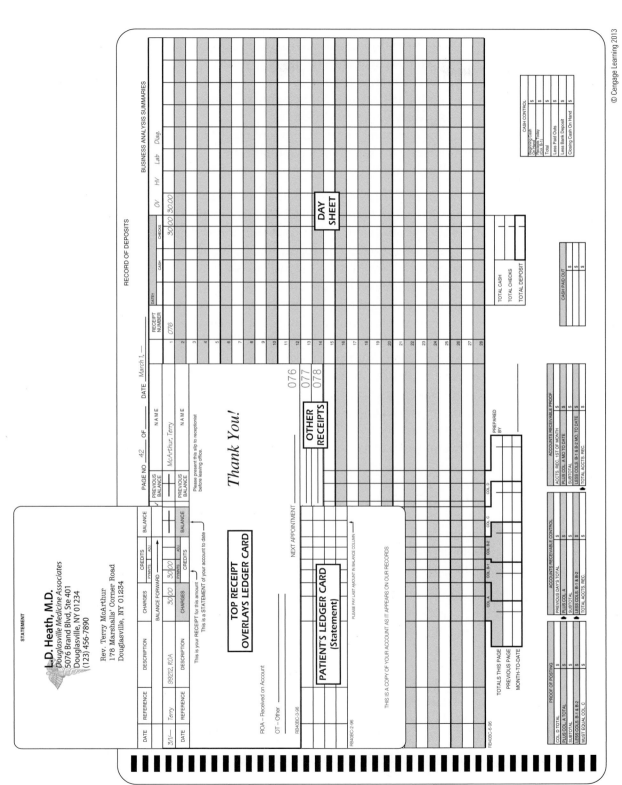

FIGURE 1-15: Posting Charges and Payments Using a Receipt.

© Cengage Learning 2013

4. Enter the amount for the service in the charge column, any adjustment amount, if applicable (discussed in **Recording Payments and Adjustments Received through the Mail),** the payment, and balance.
5. Record the type and amount of payment in the Business Analysis Summaries columns, as applicable.
6. Record the payment in the record of deposit section of the day sheet listing the entry under cash or check.
7. The receipt may be used to record the patient's next appointment, if known.
8. Remove the shingle of receipt forms from the pegboard and file the patient's ledger card.

When using a receipt, it is important to use the shingles in consecutive order as it is a security check to keep track of all receipts processed during the workday.

Always use a ballpoint pen to enter the information to be reproduced, and press firmly so that a legible copy appears on the day sheet. Occasionally check the appearance of your copy on the day sheet to make sure you are applying enough pressure when printing on the top form.

Patients are charged for services performed according to an established fee schedule that indicates the procedure code and fee charged for each type of service. The inside front and back covers include a list of codes and fees to be used in the pegboard simulation. Most patients are requested to pay by check or cash at the time services are provided, although some offices accept debit and credit card payments. Patients may also arrange to pay at a later date or to make budget payments according to the policies of the individual office. Some payments are received from third-party insurers, such as Blue Cross/Blue Shield, Medicaid, Medicare, Tricare, and other insurance carriers representing health maintenance organizations (HMOs).

Posting Charges and Payments Using a Superbill

To post or record a charge, you will need to record information simultaneously on the superbill, ledger card, and the day sheet. So, first pull the patient ledger card from the files for an established patient or prepare a ledger card for a new patient.

The steps in preparing the superbill are as follows:

1. Place the next numbered superbill on the pegboard, aligning the bottom pink layer of the superbill with the appropriate line on the day sheet, making sure that the carbon strip (Previous Balance and Name) is aligned with the first open writing line of the day sheet.
2. Insert the patient's ledger card under the pink portion of the superbill so that the first open writing line of the card is aligned with the carbon strip **(see Figure 1-16).**
3. Print the patient's previous balance and name by referring to the ledger card. Make sure you press firmly so that all information is legible on the copies of the superbill and day sheet Number 43 for March 4.
4. Enter the number of the superbill in the receipt number column.
5. Carefully flip the white and yellow layers of the superbill over to the left so that they lie flat, out of the way for recording information on the pink copy.

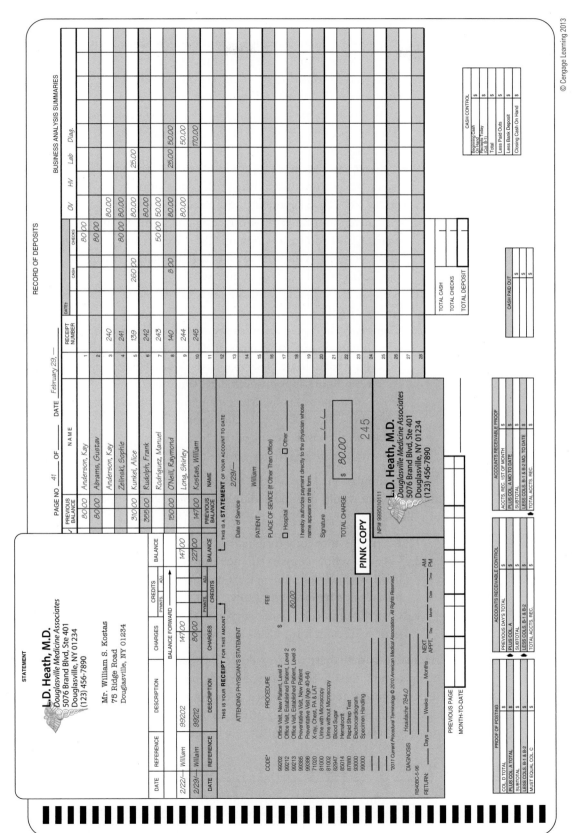

FIGURE 1-16: Posting Charges and Payments Using a Superbill.

6. Record the date in the Date column.

7. Record the patient's first name in the Reference column.

8. In the Description column, print the appropriate procedure code(s) and the abbreviation ROA (received on account if there was a payment made to the account for that visit). All procedures are coded according to the CPT code book. Look up the codes you will need for this simulation on the inside front cover of the book. Enter the charge listed for the CPT code used in the charge column.

9. If a payment was made, for example the co-pay, enter the amount in the payment column after noting in the description column *ROA pt.* Remember to record the payment in the Record of Deposit Column.

10. Calculate the Balance by subtracting any payment (if any) from today's charges, and add to any Previous Balance. In this simulation a dash is drawn in the column to indicate zeros or a zero balance; it is up to the discretion of the facility if zeros or dashes are used.

11. Remove the superbill from the pegboard, flipping the white and yellow copies back in place.

12. Complete the front section of the white copy of the superbill checking off or filling in all applicable parts of the superbill, including the individual procedure fee(s), date of service (today's date), patient's full name, total charge, and next appointment date. On the lines after "DIAGNOSIS," write the diagnosis code. Most insurance companies require the use of ICD-CM codes. The ICD-9-CM codes you will need for this simulation are found on the inside covers of this text.

13. Return the patient's ledger card to the file.

For this simulation, keep all the superbill copies together. After completing the superbill, you would distribute the three copies of the superbill **(see Figure 1-17)** as follows:

1. Keep the white copy (original) as the office file copy.

2. Give the yellow copy (insurance copy) to the patient to be attached to his or her insurance claim form. This statement contains all the information the physician is required to supply.

3. Give the pink copy (patient's personal copy) to the patient as well; the patient will retain it for his or her own record-keeping purposes.

Because a patient may often make a payment to cover the co-pay charge before being seen by the physician, a receipt may be used for this payment.

 If a computerized system is used, a receipt may be generated and printed after the transaction is posted and the patient record is updated. If the transaction is to be posted at a later time, the patient may be given a hand-written receipt.

Recording Payments and Adjustments Received Through the Mail

The procedure for recording payments received through the mail is similar to posting charges and payment as described in the previous sections, except no receipt or superbill is needed. The payment from a check received through the mail is done by

PLEASE RETURN THIS FORM TO THE RECEPTIONIST

| PREVIOUS BALANCE | NAME |

ATTENDING PHYSICIAN'S STATEMENT

Date of Service _____

PATIENT _____

PLACE OF SEVICE (If Other Than Office)

☐ Hospital _____   ☐ Other _____

I hereby authorize payment directly to the physician whose name appears on this form.

Signature _____ __/__/__

CODE*	PROCEDURE	FEE
99202	Office Visit, New Patient, Level 2	$ _____
99212	Office Visit, Established Patient, Level 2	_____
99213	Office Visit, Established Patient, Level 3	_____
99385	Preventative Visit, New Patient	_____
99386	Preventative Visit (Age 40-64)	_____
71020	X-ray, Chest, PA & LAT	_____
81000	Urine with Microscopy	_____
81002	Urine without Microscopy	_____
82947	Blood Sugar	_____
85014	Hematocrit	_____
87880	Rapid Strep Test	_____
93000	Electrocardiogram	_____
99000	Specimen Handling	_____

TOTAL CHARGE $ _____

WHITE COPY

245

2011 Current Procedural Terminology © 2010 American Medical Association. All Rights Reserved.

NPI# 9995010111

INSURANCE COPY - ATTACH THIS STATEMENT TO YOUR INSURANCE CLAIM FORM
Complete the personal information requested on the form. This statement contains all the information the insurance carrier requests of the doctor. It is not necessary for this office to fill out the insurance company claim form.

NAME

ATTENDING PHYSICIAN'S STATEMENT

Date of Service _____

PATIENT _____

PLACE OF SEVICE (If Other Than Office)

☐ Hospital _____   ☐ Other _____

I hereby authorize payment directly to the physician whose name appears on this form.

Signature _____ __/__/__

CODE*	PROCEDURE	FEE
99202	Office Visit, New Patient, Level 2	$ _____
99212	Office Visit, Established Patient, Level 2	_____
99213	Office Visit, Established Patient, Level 3	_____
99385	Preventative Visit, New Patient	_____
99386	Preventative Visit (Age 40-64)	_____
71020	X-ray, Chest, PA & LAT	_____
81000	Urine with Microscopy	_____
81002	Urine without Microscopy	_____
82947	Blood Sugar	_____
85014	Hematocrit	_____
87880	Rapid Strep Test	_____
93000	Electrocardiogram	_____
99000	Specimen Handling	_____

TOTAL CHARGE $ _____

YELLOW COPY

245

2011 Current Procedural Terminology © 2010 American Medical Association. All Rights Reserved.

NPI# 9995010111

DATE	REFERENCE	DESCRIPTION	CHARGES	PYMNTS. CREDITS	ADJ.	BALANCE	PREVIOUS BALANCE	NAME

THIS IS YOUR **RECEIPT** FOR THIS AMOUNT ___   THIS IS A **STATEMENT** OF YOUR ACCOUNT TO DATE

ATTENDING PHYSICIAN'S STATEMENT

Date of Service _____

PATIENT _____

PLACE OF SEVICE (If Other Than Office)

☐ Hospital _____   ☐ Other _____

I hereby authorize payment directly to the physician whose name appears on this form.

Signature _____ __/__/__

CODE*	PROCEDURE	FEE
99202	Office Visit, New Patient, Level 2	$ _____
99212	Office Visit, Established Patient, Level 2	_____
99213	Office Visit, Established Patient, Level 3	_____
99385	Preventative Visit, New Patient	_____
99386	Preventative Visit (Age 40-64)	_____
71020	X-ray, Chest, PA & LAT	_____
81000	Urine with Microscopy	_____
81002	Urine without Microscopy	_____
82947	Blood Sugar	_____
85014	Hematocrit	_____
87880	Rapid Strep Test	_____
93000	Electrocardiogram	_____
99000	Specimen Handling	_____

TOTAL CHARGE $ _____

PINK COPY

245

2011 Current Procedural Terminology © 2010 American Medical Association. All Rights Reserved.

NPI# 9995010111

L.D. Heath, M.D.
Douglasville Medicine Associates
5076 Brand Blvd, Ste 401
Douglasville, NY 01234
(123) 456-7890

DIAGNOSIS _____

RB40BC-5-96

RETURN: ___ Days ___ Weeks ___ Months   NEXT APPT. ___ Day ___ Month ___ Date ___ Time   AM / PM

© Cengage Learning 2013

FIGURE 1-17: White, Yellow, and Pink Copies of the Superbill.

placing the ledger card on the next available line of the day sheet and entering the transaction directly on the ledger card and day sheet simultaneously (refer back to Figure 1-14).

Patients are requested not to send cash through the mail and the patient's cancelled check serves as a receipt of payment. If the patient does send cash through the mail, many offices prepare a receipt and keep it in the patient's medical record to give to the patient at the next visit, while other offices may opt to mail the receipt to the patient.

An **adjustment** is a change made in a patient's account due to a "write-off," which is basically money the office cannot expect to collect, even if it was part of the office charge and usually occurs when a payment on an account is involved. An adjustment may occur when the office has made a legal agreement or contracted with an insurance carrier such as Medicare or Aetna to accept the payment they allow for a service provided to a member of that insurance. When a contract is signed between the insurance carrier and the **participating physician** (primary care physician [PCP]), the physician agrees to accept the fee schedule amount the insurance carrier will pay for a specific procedure code. Although the medical office charges an amount according to its own **fee schedule**, the physician must accept the insurance carrier's allowed amount as payment in full. The difference between the amount the physician charged and the insurance carrier allowed will be written off as an adjustment, meaning the physician cannot collect that amount, nor does the patient have to pay that amount; it is a "write-off."

The steps in posting a payment and an adjustment are as follows:

1. Place the ledger card over the day sheet so that the next blank line on the card aligns with the first open writing line on the day sheet. Fill in the Date and Reference columns on the ledger card.

2. In the Description column write no procedure codes; these were recorded on the day the procedures were performed. If the payment is made by the patient, print ROA in this column. The word "check" or "cash" next to the ROA can be used as a safety measure in recording the correct type of payment. If the payment is from the patient's insurer, print OT (meaning other) followed by a comma and the name of the insurance carrier such as Medicare. Enter nothing in the Charge column. Enter the amount of the payment from the insurance carrier in the "pymnts" column, and the provider adjustment discount amount listed from the Provider Explanation of Benefits (EOB) in the "adj" column on the ledger card (**see Figure 1-18**). Different insurance carriers refer to the adjustment column by various names such as the provider *adjustment discount* or the *provider's liability.* Whatever descriptive term is used for the adjustment column it means that the amount listed in that column is the amount that needs to be written off.

3. Add together the payment and the adjustment and subtract the amount from the balance due on the ledger card. This amount becomes the new balance and is recorded in the Balance column. When payments are made by a third party, usually an insurance carrier, an **Explanation of Benefits (EOB)** accompanies the payment listing the charge, the amount allowed

STATEMENT

L.D. Heath, M.D.
Douglasville Medicine Associates
5076 Brand Blvd, Ste 401
Douglasville, NY 01234
(123) 456-7890

Ms. Julie T. Fedak
53 Spring Hill Road
Douglasville, NY 01234

| DATE | REFERENCE | DESCRIPTION | CHARGES | CREDITS | | BALANCE | |
				PYMNTS.	ADJ.		
		BALANCED FORWARD ➞				527	00
2/15	Julie	OT Medicare CK		241	49	225	13	60	38

© Cengage Learning 2013

FIGURE 1-18: Posting a Payment and Adjustment.

by the insurance company and the adjustment that must be made by the participating physician, the payment made, and the amount the patient is responsible for such as a co-pay, **co-insurance**, or a **deductible.** (Terms will be discussed in further detail later in this section, in **Procedure 12 Insurance Coverage**.)

4. Because no receipt is needed, a line is drawn though the receipt column. Record the insurance payment amount in *Record of Deposit* column under checks. Do not, however, record any amounts in the *Business Analysis Summaries* columns. These amounts were recorded on the day the procedures were performed. Return the patient's ledger card to the files.

Posting a Refund

A refund may be made to either the patient or the insurance carrier when an insurance carrier paid more than expected or if the patient paid more than was required. For example, a patient may pay a co-pay for an office physical only to find out when the insurance payment arrives that a co-pay was not required for a complete physical. The medical office now has the responsibility to return the overpayment to the patient. After a payment from the patient's insurance carrier is posted and the adjustment is made for the insurance allowance, the amount paid will be more than the balance left for the service provided since the patient paid an unnecessary co-pay (**see Figure 1-19**).

STATEMENT

L.D. Heath, M.D.
Douglasville Medicine Associates
5076 Brand Blvd, Ste 401
Douglasville, NY 01234
(123) 456-7890

Mr. Javier Espinoza
11 Meadow Brook Road
Douglasville, NY 01234

DATE	REFERENCE	DESCRIPTION	CHARGES	CREDITS PYMNTS.	CREDITS ADJ.	BALANCE	
		BALANCED FORWARD ⟶				91	00
2/15	Javier	OT signal CK		111	00			<10	00>
2/15	Javier	Refund				<10	00>	———	

FIGURE 1-19: Posting a Refund.

The steps in posting a refund are as follows:

1. Place the ledger card over the day sheet so that the next blank line on the card aligns with the first open writing line on the day sheet. Fill in the Date and Reference columns on the ledger card. A receipt or superbill is not used for this procedure.

2. Do not enter procedure codes in the Description column; these were recorded on the day the procedures were performed.

3. The overpayment amount listed on the ledger card is indicated by using brackets, for example, <20> to designate a credit balance. Some offices may enter the credit balance in red ink but if the ledger card was to be copied, the red ink would not show up, so most offices use brackets to designate a credit balance. Enter nothing in the Charge column. If the refund check is going to a patient, write "Refund" in the description column. Enter nothing in the Charge column; enter the amount of the refund in the Adjustments column, putting brackets around the monetary amount of the refund. For example <20> indicating that the brackets mean to subtract and in this instance, $20 will be subtracted from the income (the previously paid amount by the patient) because it is being returned to the patient. The balance for this service is usually reduced to zero.

4. There is nothing to record in the Business Analysis Summaries columns. Return the patient's ledger card to the files.

STATEMENT

 L.D. Heath, M.D.
Douglasville Medicine Associates
5076 Brand Blvd, Ste 401
Douglasville, NY 01234
(123) 456-7890

Mrs. Jodee Pate
103 Marble Ave, Apt A
Douglasville, NY 01234

| DATE | REFERENCE | DESCRIPTION | CHARGES | CREDITS | | BALANCE | |
				PYMNTS.	ADJ.		
		BALANCED FORWARD ⟶					
2/15	Jodee	99202 ROA CK	147	00	20	00			127	00
2/25	Jodee	NSF					<20	00>	147	00

© Cengage Learning 2013

FIGURE 1-20: Posting Nonsufficient Funds (NSF).

Posting Nonsufficient Funds (NSF)

If a patient pays with a personal check that fails to clear the bank due to **nonsufficient funds (NSF),** the charge needs to be added back onto a patient's balance (**see Figure 1-20**). A notice from the bank will come to the office, stating that the check has insufficient funds and payment was denied. Most offices have a procedure in the Policy Manual for the handling of NSF. The patient is usually called for notification of the issue and the charge must then be reinstated on the ledger card.

The steps in posting an NSF check are as follows:

1. Place the ledger card over the day sheet so that the next blank line on the card aligns with the first open writing line on the day sheet. Fill in the Date and Reference columns on the ledger card. A receipt or superbill is not used for this procedure since the notification of the NSF check came through the mail.
2. There are no procedure codes to be entered in the Description column; these were recorded on the day the procedures were performed. Write "NSF" in the description column instead.
3. Add the amount of the NSF check back into the patient's account, since it can no longer be counted, as paid by entering in the Adjustment column the amount of the check in brackets (for example, <20>).
4. Add the amount of the NSF check back into the current balance column on the ledger card as well, and add in any processing charge the bank may have

levied on the medical office for processing the NSF check. Depending on state laws, the office may have the right to pass this added processing charge on to the patient, which may be described in the Description column as a miscellaneous charge. The balance for this service is usually the original charge for the service that was entered on the day of the visit and may now consist of the added bank fee that was charged to the office. An itemized statement should be sent to the patient reflecting the new balance. There is nothing to record in the Business Analysis Summaries columns. Return the patient's ledger card to the files.

Posting Entries from Collection Agencies

If the need arises to turn delinquent accounts over to a reputable collection agency (CA), the medical office no longer sends statements to the patient. Payments from the patient usually go directly to the CA, which will then send the percentage of the payment due to the physician's office. When a payment comes from the CA on a patient's account the payment and adjustment is entered on the ledger card (**see Figure 1-21**).

Most offices prefer to prevent delinquent accounts and having to send patients to a CA not only because it interferes with good will between the physician's office

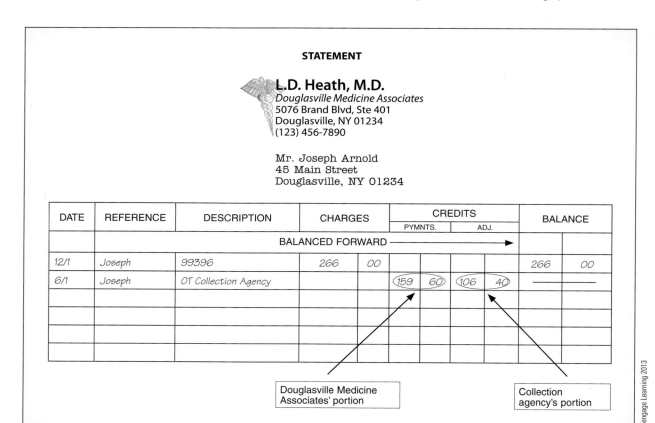

STATEMENT

L.D. Heath, M.D.
Douglasville Medicine Associates
5076 Brand Blvd, Ste 401
Douglasville, NY 01234
(123) 456-7890

Mr. Joseph Arnold
45 Main Street
Douglasville, NY 01234

DATE	REFERENCE	DESCRIPTION	CHARGES		CREDITS				BALANCE	
					PYMNTS.		ADJ.			
		BALANCED FORWARD ⟶								
12/1	Joseph	99396	266	00					266	00
6/1	Joseph	OT Collection Agency			159	60	106	40		

Douglasville Medicine Associates' portion

Collection agency's portion

© Cengage Learning 2013

FIGURE 1-21: Posting a Check from a Collection Agency.

and the patient but also because most collection agencies keep a large percentage of funds collected, decreasing the income for the physician's office.

The steps in posting a payment from a CA are as follows:

1. Place the ledger card over the day sheet so that the next blank line on the card aligns with the first open writing line on the day sheet. Fill in the Date and Reference columns on the ledger card. A receipt or superbill is not used for this procedure.
2. No procedure codes are entered in the Description column; these were recorded on the day the procedures were performed. Write "ROA from CA" in the Description column.
3. Enter the amount of the payment received from the CA in the Payments column and enter the adjustment amount listed on the EOB from the CA, which typically can be 22% to 45% of the original charge. The balance for this date of service is usually zero, and the account from the CA is closed.

Payments by Direct Deposit

Notification of direct deposit payments usually come with the insurance carrier's EOB and many times the check will be payment for a number of patient accounts. The posting procedures are the same as if the check came in the mail from an individual, with each patient account receiving the amount paid for a specific date of service. Care must be taken that the total amount of the check adds up correctly after entering all payments for individual patients.

Posting Hospital Charges

Hospital charges can be added to a ledger card in a few different ways, according to the policy of the office. In this simulation, you will enter all the charges on one line and the total charge will be the sum of the admission, the daily visits, and the discharge visit.

The steps to post the hospital charges for a patient admitted on 2/15 and discharged on 2/18 are:

1. Place the patient's ledger card on the next available line of the day sheet.
2. Enter the dates of the hospitalization (2/15–2/18) in the DATE column.
3. Enter the name of the patient in the REFERENCE column.
4. In the DESCRIPTION column enter the CPT code for a hospital admission (99221). Write the amount of the charge ($145.00) on a separate piece of paper.
5. Enter the daily visit code on the same line (99231) on the ledger card. There are two daily visits, one for 2/16 and one for 2/17. Add to the admission charge two daily visit charges ($79.00 × 2 days = $158.00). On the insurance claim form, you would enter the charge amount ($79.00) in column 24F, the charge column; in column 24G, enter 2. This information

STATEMENT

L.D. Heath, M.D.
Douglasville Medicine Associates
5076 Brand Blvd, Ste 401
Douglasville, NY 01234
(123) 456-7890

Mrs. Fiona J. Markham
2 State Street
Douglasville, NY 01234

DATE	REFERENCE	DESCRIPTION	CHARGES	CREDITS		BALANCE	
				PYMNTS.	ADJ.		
		BALANCED FORWARD ———————————————➤					
2/15–2/18	Fiona	99221 99231 99238	448	00			448	00

FIGURE 1-22: Posting Hospital Charges.

tells the insurance carrier that the daily hospital visit charge is $79 and the "2" means that this charge is $79 × 2 days. The insurance carrier wants to see the itemized per day charges in these columns.

6. Finally, on the ledger card, enter the discharge visit date on the same line and add the charge to the admission and daily visit charges. Place the total amount in the Charge column (**see Figure 1-22**).

PROCEDURE 8: TOTALING THE DAY SHEET

The day sheet (record of charges and receipts) is used to keep track of patient accounts. It contains a running total of **accounts receivable,** the total balance due from patients for services rendered by the physician (**see Figure 1-23**). The day sheet informs the physician of the amount of money collected that day and the amount still owed.

Proof of Posting

Each day, all columns of the day sheet should be totaled and proved. Proving the totals involves verifying their correctness once added. By proving the totals daily, you can correct errors immediately before they are carried over into the next day. Because errors are costly, minimizing them is an important part of your job.

DAY SHEET (RECORD OF CHARGES AND RECEIPTS)   PAGE NO 23 OF ___   DATE February 2

DATE	REFERENCE	DESCRIPTION	CHARGES		CREDITS			BALANCE		√	PREVIOUS BALANCE		NAME
					PYMNTS.	ADJ.							
2/2	Arlene	07 Blue Shield			65 00			40 00			105 00		Billings, Arlene
2/2	Godfrey	07 Statewide			72 00	8 00		—			80 00		Singh, Godfrey
2/2	Carmen	99202 ROA CK	147 00		147 00			—			—		Sanchez, Carmen
2/2	Anne	99212 ROA CK	80 00		110 00			—			30 00		Drake, Anne
2/2	Tyrone	99213 93000 ROA cash	142 00		20 00			152 00			30 00		Brooks, Tyrone
2/2	Michael	99212 ROA CK	80 00		320 00			—			240 00		Ryan, Michael
2/2	Ki	99396	266 00					266 00			—		Kim, Ki

RECORD OF DEPOSITS   BUSINESS ANALYSIS SUMARIES

RECEIPT NUMBER	CASH		CHECKS		OV	HV	LAB	DIAG
1			65	00	00			
2			72	00	00			
3			147	00	147			
4			110	00	80			
5	20	00			111			
6			320	00	80			
7					266			
8								
9								
10								
11								
12								
13								
14								
15								
16								
17								
18								
19								
20								
21								
22								
23								
24								
25								
26								
27								
28					684			131

	Col A		Col. B-1		Col. B-2		Col. C		Col. D	
	715	00	734	00	8	00	458	00	485	00
	955	00	816	00	0		525	00	386	00
	1670	00	1550	00	8	00	983	00	871	00

TOTALS THIS PAGE
PREVIOUS PAGE
MONTH-TO-DATE

TOTAL CASH	20	00
TOTAL CHECKS	714	00
TOTAL DEPOSIT	734	00

CASH CONTROL		
Beginning Cash On Hand	$	36.50
Receipts Today (Col. B-1)	$	734.00
Total $		770.00
Less Paid Outs		4.30
Less Bank Deposit		734.00
Closing Cash On Hand	$	32.20

Prepared By _____

CASH PAID OUT	
	$ 2.45
	$ 1.85
	$

PROOF OF POSTING		
COL. D TOTAL	$	485.00
PLUS COL.A TOTAL	$	715.00
SUB TOTAL	$	1,200.00
LESS COLS.B1 &B-2	$	742.00
MUST EQUAL COL.C	$	458.00

ACCOUNTS RECEIVABLE CONTROL		
PREVIOUS DAY'S TOTAL	$	2,184.00
PLUS COLA	$	715.00
SUB TOTAL	$	2,899.00
LESS COLS. B-1 &B-2	$	742.00
TOTAL ACCTS. REC	$	2,157.00

ACCOUNTS RECEIVABLE PROOF		
ACCTS. REC. 1ST OF MONTH	$	2,045.00
PLUS COLA MONTH TO DATE	$	1,670.00
SUB TOTAL	$	3,715.00
LESS B-1 & B-2 MO. TO DATE	$	1,558.00
TOTAL ACCTS. REC	$	2,157.00

FIGURE 1-23: Totaling the Day Sheet.

Near the bottom of the day sheet are the totals for the day (Totals This Page). To obtain these totals just add all figures in that column. On the next line, carry over that column's totals from the previous page. For example, when setting up the day sheet for Tuesday, March 5, the Month-To-Date totals from Monday, March 4, would be carried over and placed in the "Previous Page" column on March 5. This procedure allows the pegboard system to keep a running total of the charges, income, adjustment, and current balance throughout the month. After you have proved today's totals (see the next three paragraphs), add these lines together to get the total for the month-to-date.

The Proof of Posting box at the bottom left side of the day sheet is used to verify that the totals have been added and posted correctly for the day. Fill in the figures as indicated and add or subtract as required. The amount in the last line of the Proof of Posting box must equal the top line of Column C in the Totals This Page. If the two amounts are equal, it means that you have verified that the current balance equals the previous balance plus all charges and minus all payments and adjustments for the day. You are now ready to move on to the middle box.

Accounts Receivable Control

The middle box is the Accounts Receivable Control box. Fill in the figures and perform the calculations requested. This box indicates that the day's charges are added to and the day's payments are subtracted from the previous balance. This gives the physician the new total of accounts receivable for the month.

Accounts Receivable Proof

The next box, the Accounts Receivable Proof box, takes the total at the beginning of this month (Total Accounts Receivable figure from the last day sheet of last month) and adds all charges and subtracts all payments and adjustments for the month to give the new total of accounts receivable. The number in the bottom line of this box must be the same number as in the last line of the preceding box, the Accounts Receivable Control box. If the figures do not match, recheck the entries and the calculations.

You may want to choose a time when you are free from distractions to do these calculations. More errors occur when someone is tired and rushed so an office may leave the day sheet calculations to the following morning. Computing the calculations on a separate sheet of paper before entering them in pen on the day sheet is advisable in order to keep the record legible.

Cash Paid Out and Cash Control (Petty Cash)

The Cash Paid Out box is used to keep track of **petty cash**. Sometimes expenses occur in the office that requires small amounts of cash, such as postage due. Any cash spent is recorded as cash paid out. Each facility determines the amount of cash needed for minor expenses. Each time an employee uses any money from the petty cash fund for miscellaneous expenses, a voucher is filled out listing the date, the reason for the cash need, and the person's name who withdrew the cash. When the petty cash fund is getting low the vouchers are collected and turned in to the employee responsible for writing checks. A check is written and cashed for the amount of money used and the cash is returned to the petty cash fund. Any cash left at the office should be locked up for security reasons at the end of the day.

The Cash Control box keeps track of cash (all monies) in the office. Record the Beginning Cash on Hand (Closing Cash on Hand figure from previous page) and add the total of all receipts for the day. Subtract both the cash paid out and the daily deposit. This amount is the Closing Cash on Hand which will be the Beginning Cash on Hand for the next day.

Business Analysis Summaries

The Business Analysis Summaries section is used by the accounting firm to advise the physician about office costs. This section of the day sheet can help facilities determine the cost effectiveness of various procedures or simply the amount of payment generated by specific procedures. It is customized for individual facilities, or may not even be used at all. In this simulation, the Douglasville Medicine Associates practice is monitoring the amount of revenue generated from office visits, hospital visits, laboratory work, and diagnostic procedures. If, for example, the laboratory revenue is very high, the practice might be advised that it would be advantageous to expand the laboratory to meet the increased demands of patients. If the revenue was very low, it might be better to close the laboratory and send all patients elsewhere for laboratory testing. Information for the Business Analysis Section is gathered as the patients are processed throughout the office and may be totaled at the end of the day to evaluate what services are used most often.

Record of Deposits

Deposits should be made daily because a large amount of money should not be left in the office overnight for security reasons. Some pegboard systems provide a detachable deposit sheet on the day sheet that makes totaling up the deposit slip convenient with less chance of error due to rewriting the amount to be deposited. Other pegboard systems use the information from the day sheet to prepare the deposit slip. Before checks are deposited, they must be endorsed.

Check Endorsements

Two commonly used types of check endorsements are **blank endorsement** and **restrictive endorsement**. A *blank endorsement* has a signature only on the back of a check, which allows anyone who signs the check to cash it. A lost or stolen check might be cashed if measures were not taken to prevent this from occurring.

A *restrictive endorsement* (**see Figure 1-24**) prevents anyone other than the endorser, the person for whom the check is intended, from cashing the check. A

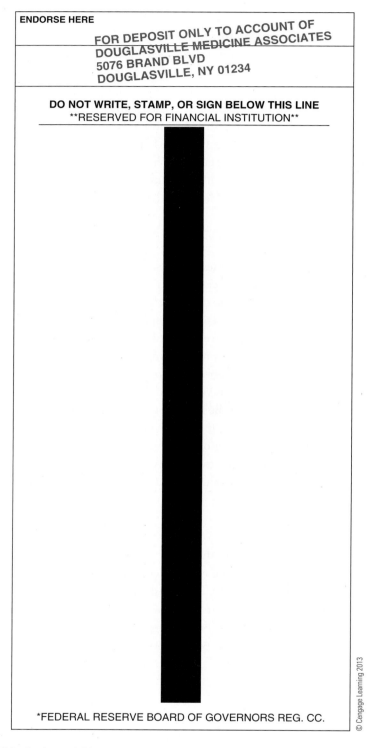

FIGURE 1-24: Endorsed Check.

customized endorsement stamp for the office with words—for example, *for deposit only to the account of Douglasville Medicine Associates 5076 Brand Blvd, Douglasville, NY 01234* should be used on the back of each check as it arrives in the office to guard against having it stolen or lost and illegally cashed. All checks should be examined for proper endorsement prior to deposit. Many offices have a policy regarding accepting third-party checks other than from insurance carriers. Be sure that any check accepted is properly dated, has the correct amount written, and is properly signed. Toward the end of each workday, you will prepare a deposit slip that lists all cash and checks being deposited. In this simulation, another employee takes care of depositing the money with The First National Bank.

Preparing the Deposit Slip

Total the Cash and Checks columns on the day sheet to determine the daily deposit amount. Each day, Douglasville Medicine Associates follows the common practice of depositing all cash and checks on hand. One of your responsibilities as the medical office professional is to safeguard all cash and checks received and to prepare the daily deposit ticket (**see Figure 1-25**).

1. Enter the date of deposit.
2. Count all cash on hand to make sure that the amount of bills and coins agrees with the receipts recorded in the Cash column of the day sheet. Arrange bills in order and facing the same direction. Enter in the currency box on the deposit slip. Count any coins and add the total to the coins section on the deposit slip. If a large number of coins were collected, they may need to be rolled before depositing them. Record the amount on the deposit slip.
3. Be sure that the back of each check is properly endorsed.
4. List all checks to be deposited by writing the amount of the check clearly on the deposit slip following the deposit policy of the bank.
5. Add and record the total of all cash and checks on the deposit slip.
6. Enter the total deposit in the check register. (See Procedure 9: Completing the Check Register.)

PROCEDURE 9: COMPLETING THE CHECK REGISTER

The check register, another part of the pegboard system, serves as a record of checks issued and as a cash disbursements journal for **accounts payable**, the balance due to creditors for supplies and services purchased by the physician. Special checks and forms designed for the pegboard system are used for the accounts payable section and are customized for the individual physician's office. A check register and the necessary checks are provided for this simulation.

To begin using the check register, remove all forms from the pegboard. Attach the check register form, placing the top hole of the sheet over the top peg. At the top left, identify the sheet recording the month and year of your first transaction on this sheet. In an office situation you would also fill in the next consecutive page number. Use the shingle of checks provided for the pegboard to complete the checks.

DEPOSIT TICKET

TO INSURE CLEAR COPY PRESS FIRMLY ON PEN
USE THIS TICKET FOR ALL DEPOSITS ENDORSE ALL CHECKS
WHEN MAILING DEPOSIT, PLEASE PRINT OR TYPE ADDRESS

DATE *February 2, —*

		DOLLARS	CENTS
BILLS		20	00
COIN			
CHECK	1	65	00
	2	72	00
	3	147	00
	4	110	00
	5	320	00
	6		
	7		
	8		
	9		
	10		
	11		
	12		
	13		
	14		
	15		
	16		
	17		
	18		
	19		
	20		
TOTAL		734	00

FOR BANK USE

CHECKS AND OTHER ITEMS ARE RECIEVED FOR DEPOSIT SUBJECT TO THE PROVISIONS OF THE UNIFORM COMMERCIAL CODE OR ANY APPLICABLE COLLECTION AGREEMENT

LISA MARTINEZ, M.D.
420 Broad Street
Hopewell, NJ 08525

FOR INSTRUCTIONAL USE ONLY

THE FIRST NATIONAL BANK
Princeton, NJ 08540-2222

3-2/310

⑆031000059⑆ 170⑈916 3⑈

FIGURE 1-25: Preparing the Deposit Slip.

Distribution Columns

A pegboard check register system is used for disbursements **(see Figure 1-26)**.

Write the following headings at the top of the Expense Disbursement columns. In this simulation, beginning with Medical Supplies in box 1 and ending with Net Payroll in box 15. Fold the form over to complete all entries. For convenience, Column 11 will be left blank, and the payroll information will be put in Columns 12–15.

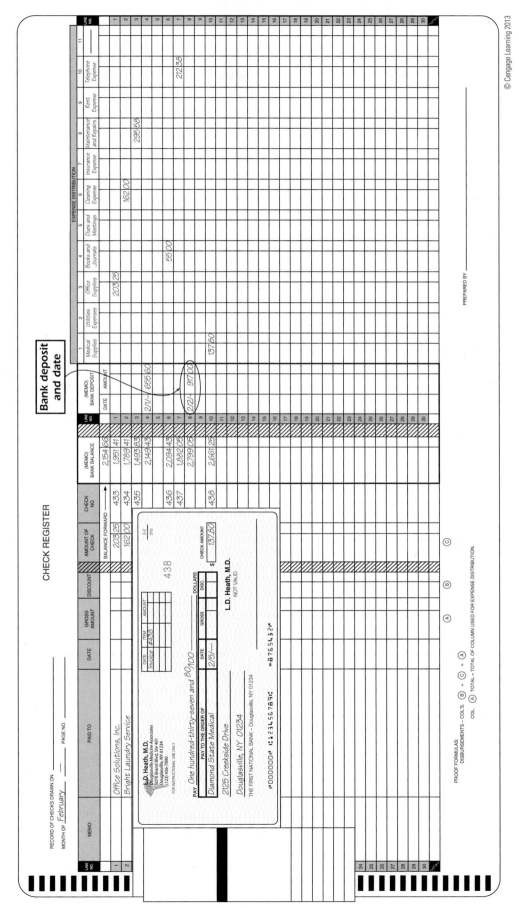

FIGURE 1-26: Check Register.

1. Medical Supplies
2. Utilities Expenses
3. Office Supplies
4. Books and Journals
5. Dues and Meetings
6. Cleaning Expenses
7. Insurance Expenses
8. Maintenance and Repairs
9. Rent Expenses
10. Telephone Expenses
11. Federal Withholding
12. State Withholding
13. Social Security (SS) and Medicare
14. Net Payroll
15. Miscellaneous

These headings are the names of expense accounts used by the accounting service that prepares Douglasville Medicine Associates' financial statements. In the Description box under Miscellaneous, write "Tax Returns." You will use the category in the simulation to record a payment to the accounting service. The columns numbered 16 through 22 will not be used in the simulation. This simulation has provided column expenses for you to use although the columns may be customized for each medical facility. As each check is prepared, enter the amount under the appropriate distribution column. The check register sheet also allows you to break down the various kinds of expenses incurred by the medical office. Each expenditure is classified by recording the amount of the check written in the appropriate expense disbursement column. With each deposit you make and each check you write, you will recalculate the bank balance. At any time, therefore, your physician-employer may check on the current balance of his or her checking account.

Entering the Deposit

In the check register, locate the last line used to record a check. On the next blank line in the Bank Deposit column, write the date of the deposit and the total amount of the deposit. Add this total to the previous bank balance in the check register and record the sum on this line in the Bank Balance column. (Refer back to Figure 1-26.)

Purchase Order Responsibility

As a medical office professional, you will have several responsibilities concerning the purchasing of goods and services. In many offices you will be required to inventory and order office supplies such as copy paper, ink/toner, or patient gowns, as needed. Each office will have procedures to follow when preparing and ordering supplies.

When items are delivered, you will check the goods received against your purchase order and the **packing slip** from the supplier to be sure the order is correct. The packing slip lists only the items shipped and does not list the price of each item. The **invoice (IV)** containing the amount owed is sent through the mail. When the

Douglasville Medicine Associates
5076 Brand Blvd
Douglasville, NY 01234

Diamond State Medical

2125 Creekside Drive
Newark, DE 19711
(302) 444-9908

Invoice No.: **3256**

paid
CK #438
2/5/—
$137.80

Account No.: **270-54**
Statement Date: 1/30/—

QTY.	UNIT	CAT. NUMBER	DESCRIPTION	UNIT PRICE	AMOUNT
1	100/BX	GS243653	Sterile gloves	30.00	30.00
5	100/BX	PD895450	Patient drapes	14.00	70.00
5	100/BX	GN124360	Non-sterile gloves	6.00	30.00
			Subtotal		$130.00
			State Tax (6%)		7.80
			Total—Pay this Amount		$137.80

© Cengage Learning 2013

FIGURE 1-27: Paid Invoice.

invoice arrives it is checked against the packing slip to be sure all items ordered were received before submitting the invoice to be paid.

As invoices are received from creditors, you will file them alphabetically by the creditor's name in an unpaid bills file. As you pay each creditor, mark the invoice "Paid," recording the check number, the date of payment, and the amount of payment on each invoice, as shown in **Figure 1-27**. File the invoices alphabetically in a paid bills file. In this simulation, you should verify the accuracy of the calculations on each invoice.

Writing Checks

Accuracy is essential when preparing checks and maintaining the balance of the check register. A carbon strip on the back of each check allows you to record simultaneously on the check itself and on the check register the following information:

- Name of the payee
- Date of the check
- Amount of the check

A memo box is provided on each check as a place to enter the invoice number (IV#) or to list a reason why the check was written, such as "staff dues."

Follow these steps as you use the pegboard system's check register to complete checks in this simulation:

1. Place the shingle of prenumbered checks over the pegs, making sure that the carbon strip of the *bottom* check (earliest number) aligns with the first open writing line of the check register. When changing to a new shingle of checks, be sure to keep them in consecutive order.

2. Flip the remaining checks to the left so that they lie flat, out of the way for recording the first check.

3. Using ink, print words and figures for the amount of the check immediately after the word *Pay*—for example, "One hundred thirty-seven and 80/100." Add a horizontal line from the end of *100* to the word *dollars*. Be sure to press firmly with a ballpoint pen.

4. Print the name of the payee in the Pay to the Order Of box. Print the address on the lines below. Print the entire address at this time so that the check can be inserted into a window envelope. (Window envelopes are not provided with this simulation.)

5. Record the date (in mm/dd/yy style) and the check amount in numeric form, for example, "2/5/—" and "137.80," or 137. 80/100 (**see Figure 1-28**).

6. Record the check number in the check register.

7. Subtract the amount of the check from the bank balance on the line above to obtain the up-to-date bank balance. (Deposits are always recorded at the end of the day, in the Bank Deposit column. After recording a deposit, add the amount to the previous balance. This will be the balance from which the next check is deducted.) Double-check your calculations.

8. Record the amount of the check in the appropriate distribution column. When each expenditure is classified according to the type of expense incurred, the physician can analyze costs and exercise control over expenditures.

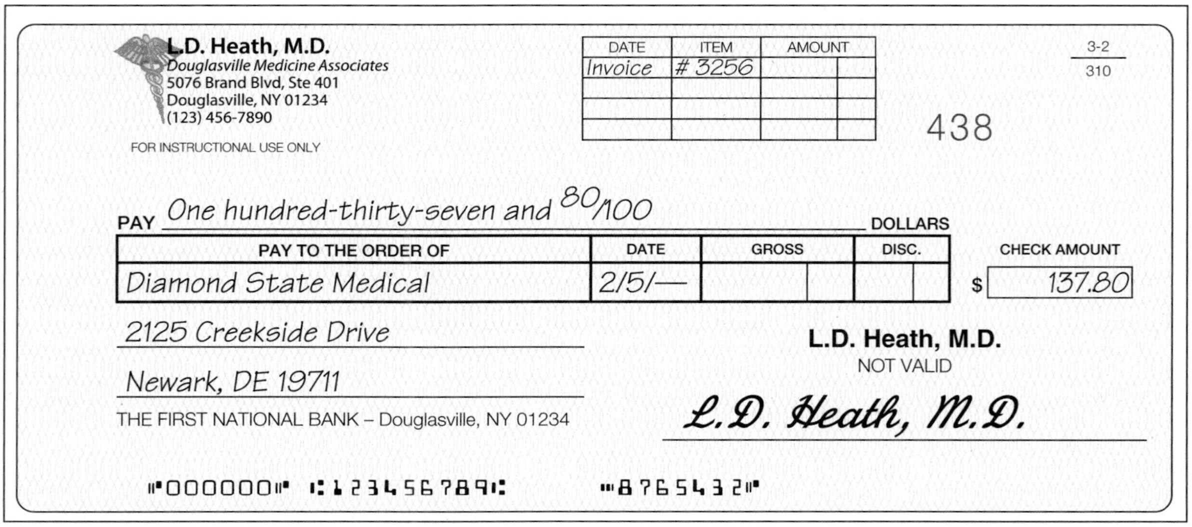

FIGURE 1-28: Completed Check.

9. Mark the invoice "Paid," recording the check number, the date, and the amount paid on each invoice. Writing the amount paid on the invoice is important because the entire bill may not be paid if some items were not received due to a back order or were to be returned.
10. Remove the check, presenting it with the related invoice to the physician for his or her signature. For the purposes of this simulation, place all completed checks in the envelope with your receipt and statement forms.

In this simulation, all bookkeeping operations that involve accounts payable, with the exception of the preparation of checks to creditors and employees, are handled by Englewood Accounting Services. This firm is responsible for preparing and filing all state and federal tax returns and for preparing semiannual and annual financial statements. You will prepare the weekly payroll for one full-time and one part-time employee.

PROCEDURE 10: PREPARING PAYROLL CHECKS TO INCLUDE WITHHOLDING

Processing payroll may be the responsibility of a medical office professional. Certain information must be gathered by new employees and reviewed each year in order to prepare accurate payroll checks. A W-2 form, a wage and tax statement **(see Figure 1-29)**,

22222 | Void ☐ | a Employee's social security number | For Official Use Only ▶ OMB No. 1545-0008

b Employer identification number (EIN)	1 Wages, tips, other compensation	2 Federal income tax withheld
c Employer's name, address, and ZIP code	3 Social security wages	4 Social security tax withheld
	5 Medicare wages and tips	6 Medicare tax withheld
	7 Social security tips	8 Allocated tips
d Control number	9 Advance EIC payment	10 Dependent care benefits
e Employee's first name and initial / Last name / Suff.	11 Nonqualified plans	12a See instructions for box 12 (Code)
	13 Statutory employee ☐ Retirement plan ☐ Third-party sick pay ☐	12b (Code)
	14 Other	12c (Code)
f Employee's address and ZIP code		12d (Code)

15 State	Employer's state ID number	16 State wages, tips, etc.	17 State income tax	18 Local wages, tips, etc.	19 Local income tax	20 Locality name

Form **W-2** Wage and Tax Statement 20__

Department of the Treasury—Internal Revenue Service

For Privacy Act and Paperwork Reduction Act Notice, see back of Copy D.

Cat. No. 10134D

Copy A For Social Security Administration — Send this entire page with Form W-3 to the Social Security Administration; photocopies are **not** acceptable.

Do Not Cut, Fold, or Staple Forms on This Page — Do Not Cut, Fold, or Staple Forms on This Page

U.S. Department of the Treasury, Internal Revenue Service.

FIGURE 1-29: W-2 Wage and Tax Statement.

is prepared by the employer and sent to each employee and the Internal Revenue Service (IRS) by the end of January, summarizing and reporting an employee's wages and payroll tax deductions for the year. A W-4 form **(see Figure 1-30)** is a form completed by the employee and given to the employer for withholding purposes. A W-4 form determines the amount of tax that will be withheld from an employee's paycheck and is based on the number of dependents, jobs, and marital status. Withholdings claimed on W-4 forms may be changed and updated each year by the employee. Payroll tax deductions are based on the employee's number of exemptions and any additional withholding amounts. The Federal Insurance Contribution Act (FICA) imposes taxes on both the employer and the employee to help fund Social Security and Medicare, programs that benefit retirees, disabled individuals, and children of deceased workers. Once the deduction amount is calculated, it is deducted from the gross wage. Accurate records must be kept of all deductions made for the payroll. The check register provides columns to keep a record of each deduction per paycheck. Any taxes due to the federal and state government are then forwarded by the employer to the correct governmental agencies. The pages needed for this simulation are provided from the *Circular E, Employer's Tax Guide* **(see Figure 1-31)** and the *State Withholding Tax Table and Methods–NY State* **(see Figure 1-32).**

The steps involved in preparing a weekly payroll check are as follows:

1. To figure the gross pay for employees, multiply the hourly salary by the hours worked per pay period. (For example, 40 hours at $15.00 per hour for a weekly pay period would be $600.00.)
2. To figure the deductions from an employee's wages, a **W4 Form** (Withholding Allowance Certification) is used; for example, **Figure 1-30** Employee's W-4 shows a married person claiming two exemptions.
3. The method used for figuring federal withholding taxes is to find the gross wages or pay in the correct wage bracket table as shown in **Figure 1-31** Circular E, Employer's Tax Guide: Federal Tax Table for Married Taxpayers, Weekly Payroll Period. For a married person with two withholding allowances who are paid $600.00 weekly, the allowance value is $20.30. State tax deductions are found in Withholding Tax Tables and Methods booklet provided by each state. In the New York State Withholding Tax Table booklet, an employee with two exemptions earning a weekly gross wage of $600.00 would have a deduction of $21.30. (Refer back to Figure 1-32, State Withholding Tax Table and Methods–NY State.)
4. FICA, or Federal Insurance Contribution Act, is a law that requires a certain amount of money to be withheld from an employee's wages for Social Security benefits. The employee pays half of the required contribution and the employer pays the other half. The Social Security benefit rate is figured by multiplying the gross wage by 6.2%. For example, if the worker earned $600.00 per week, the Social Security benefits amount deducted from the payroll would be 600×0.062 (6.2%) = $37.20.
5. The Medicare deduction is figured by multiplying the gross wage by 1.45%. For example, for the person making $600.00, the amount would be $8.70.
6. Requested deductions taken from an employee's gross wages may include health insurance, dental and vision coverage, retirement fund, or savings plan. These deductions would also be deducted from the gross wage.

Form W-4 —

Want More Money In Your Paycheck?
If you expect to be able to take the earned income credit for 19— and a child lives with you, you may be able to have part of the credit added to your take-home pay. For details, get Form W-5 from your employer.

Purpose. Complete Form W-4 so that your employer can withhold the correct amount of Federal income tax from your pay.

Exemption From Withholding. Read line 7 of the certificate below to see if you can claim exempt status. *If exempt, complete line 7; but do not complete lines 5 and 6.* No Federal income tax will be withheld from your pay. Your exemption is good for 1 year only. It expires February 15, —.

Note: *You cannot claim exemption from withholding if (1) your income exceeds $650 and includes unearned income (e.g., interest*

and dividends) and (2) another person can claim you as a dependent on their tax return.

Basic Instructions. Employees who are not exempt should complete the Personal Allowances Worksheet. Additional worksheets are provided on page 2 for employees to adjust their withholding allowances based on itemized deductions, adjustments to income, or two-earner/two-job situations. Complete all worksheets that apply to your situation. The worksheets will help you figure the number of withholding allowances you are entitled to claim. However, you may claim fewer allowances than this.

Head of Household. Generally, you may claim head of household filing status on your tax return only if you are unmarried and pay more than 50% of the costs of keeping up a home for yourself and your dependent(s) or other qualifying individuals.

Nonwage Income. If you have a large amount of nonwage income, such as interest or dividends, you should consider making

estimated tax payments using Form 1040-ES. Otherwise, you may find that you owe additional tax at the end of the year.

Two Earners/Two Jobs. If you have a working spouse or more than one job, figure the total number of allowances you are entitled to claim on all jobs using worksheets from only one Form W-4. This total should be divided among all jobs. Your withholding will usually be most accurate when all allowances are claimed on the W-4 filed for the highest paying job and zero allowances are claimed for the others.

Check Your Withholding. After your W-4 takes effect, you can use **Pub. 919**, Is My Withholding Correct for —?, to see how the dollar amount you are having withheld compares to your estimated total annual tax. We recommend you get Pub. 919 especially if you used the Two Earner/Two Job Worksheet and your earnings exceed $150,000 (Single) or $200,000 (Married). Call 1-800-829-3676 to order Pub. 919. Check your telephone directory for the IRS assistance number for further help.

Personal Allowances Worksheet

A   Enter "1" for **yourself** if no one else can claim you as a dependent . . . . **A** ___1___

B   Enter "1" if: { • You are single and have only one job; or
• You are married, have only one job, and your spouse does not work; or
• Your wages from a second job or your spouse's wages (or the total of both) are $1,000 or less. } . . **B** _____

C   Enter "1" for your **spouse**. But, you may choose to enter -0- if you are married and have either a working spouse or more than one job (this may help you avoid having too little tax withheld) . . . . **C** _____

D   Enter number of **dependents** (other than your spouse or yourself) you will claim on your tax return . . . . **D** _____

E   Enter "1" if you will file as **head of household** on your tax return (see conditions under **Head of Household** above) . **E** _____

F   Enter "1" if you have at least $1,500 of **child or dependent care expenses** for which you plan to claim a credit . . **F** _____

G   Add lines A through F and enter total here. **Note:** This amount may be different from the number of exemptions you claim on your return ▶ **G** ___1___

For accuracy, do all worksheets that apply. { • If you plan to **itemize** or claim **adjustments to income** and want to reduce your withholding, see the Deductions and Adjustments Worksheet on page 2.
• If you are **single** and have **more than one job** and your combined earnings from all jobs exceed $30,000 OR if you are **married** and have a **working spouse or more than one job**, and the combined earnings from all jobs exceed $50,000, see the Two-Earner/Two-Job Worksheet on page 2 if you want to avoid having too little tax withheld.
• If **neither** of the above situations applies, **stop here** and enter the number from line G on line 5 of Form W-4 below. }

-------------- **Cut here and give the certificate to your employer. Keep the top portion for your records.** --------------

Form **W-4** Department of the Treasury Internal Revenue Service	**Employee's Withholding Allowance Certificate** ▶ **For Privacy Act and Paperwork Reduction Act Notice, see reverse.**	OMB No. 1545-0010

1 Type or print your first name and middle initial *JOSEPH M*	Last name *PINELLI*	2 Your social security number *555 : 18 : 7218*

Home address (number and street or rural route) *4201 Gateway Boulevard*	3 ☒ Single ☐ Married ☐ Married, but withhold at higher Single rate. **Note:** *If married, but legally separated, or spouse is a nonresident alien, check the Single box.*
City or town, state, and ZIP code *Douglasville, NY 01234*	4 If your last name differs from that on your social security card, check here and call 1-800-772-1213 for a new card . . . . . ▶ ☐

5	Total number of allowances you are claiming (from line G above or from the worksheets on page 2 if they apply) .	**5**	*1*
6	Additional amount, if any, you want withheld from each paycheck	**6** $	

7   I claim exemption from withholding for 1995 and I certify that I meet **BOTH** of the following conditions for exemption:
• Last year I had a right to a refund of **ALL** Federal income tax withheld because I had **NO** tax liability; **AND**
• This year I expect a refund of **ALL** Federal income tax withheld because I expect to have **NO** tax liability.
If you meet both conditions, enter "EXEMPT" here . . . . ▶ **7** [shaded]

Under penalties of perjury, I certify that I am entitled to the number of withholding allowances claimed on this certificate or entitled to claim exempt status.

Employee's signature ▶ *Joseph M Pinelli*   Date ▶ *April 14*   , —

8 Employer's name and address (Employer: Complete 8 and 10 only if sending to the IRS)	9 Office code (optional)	10 Employer identification number

Cat. No. 10220Q

U.S. Department of the Treasury, Internal Revenue Service.

FIGURE 1-30: Employee's W-4 Form.

MARRIED Persons—**WEEKLY** Payroll Period

(For Wages Paid Through December 20__)

And the wages are–		And the number of withholding allowances claimed is—										
At least	But less than	0	1	2	3	4	5	6	7	8	9	10
		The amount of income tax to be withheld is—										
$0	$270	$0	$0	$0	$0	$0	$0	$0	$0	$0	$0	$0
270	280	1	0	0	0	0	0	0	0	0	0	0
280	290	2	0	0	0	0	0	0	0	0	0	0
290	300	3	0	0	0	0	0	0	0	0	0	0
300	310	4	0	0	0	0	0	0	0	0	0	0
310	320	5	0	0	0	0	0	0	0	0	0	0
320	330	6	0	0	0	0	0	0	0	0	0	0
330	340	7	0	0	0	0	0	0	0	0	0	0
340	350	8	1	0	0	0	0	0	0	0	0	0
350	360	9	2	0	0	0	0	0	0	0	0	0
360	370	10	3	0	0	0	0	0	0	0	0	0
370	380	11	4	0	0	0	0	0	0	0	0	0
380	390	12	5	0	0	0	0	0	0	0	0	0
390	400	13	6	0	0	0	0	0	0	0	0	0
400	410	14	7	0	0	0	0	0	0	0	0	0
410	420	15	8	1	0	0	0	0	0	0	0	0
420	430	16	9	2	0	0	0	0	0	0	0	0
430	440	17	10	3	0	0	0	0	0	0	0	0
440	450	18	11	4	0	0	0	0	0	0	0	0
450	460	19	12	5	0	0	0	0	0	0	0	0
460	470	20	13	6	0	0	0	0	0	0	0	0
470	480	21	14	7	0	0	0	0	0	0	0	0
480	490	23	15	8	1	0	0	0	0	0	0	0
490	500	24	16	9	2	0	0	0	0	0	0	0
500	510	26	17	10	3	0	0	0	0	0	0	0
510	520	27	18	11	4	0	0	0	0	0	0	0
520	530	29	19	12	5	0	0	0	0	0	0	0
530	540	30	20	13	6	0	0	0	0	0	0	0
540	550	32	21	14	7	0	0	0	0	0	0	0
550	560	33	23	15	8	1	0	0	0	0	0	0
560	570	35	24	16	9	2	0	0	0	0	0	0
570	580	36	26	17	10	3	0	0	0	0	0	0
580	590	38	27	18	11	4	0	0	0	0	0	0
590	600	39	29	19	12	5	0	0	0	0	0	0
600	610	41	30	20	13	6	0	0	0	0	0	0
610	620	42	32	21	14	7	0	0	0	0	0	0
620	630	44	33	23	15	8	1	0	0	0	0	0
630	640	45	35	24	16	9	2	0	0	0	0	0
640	650	47	36	26	17	10	3	0	0	0	0	0
650	660	48	38	27	18	11	4	0	0	0	0	0
660	670	50	39	29	19	12	5	0	0	0	0	0

FIGURE 1-31: Sample Page from *Circular E, Employer's Tax Guide.*

670	680	51	41	30	20	13	6	0	0	0	0	0
680	690	53	42	32	21	14	7	0	0	0	0	0
690	700	54	44	33	23	15	8	1	0	0	0	0
700	710	56	45	35	24	16	9	2	0	0	0	0
710	720	57	47	36	26	17	10	3	0	0	0	0
720	730	59	48	38	27	18	11	4	0	0	0	0
730	740	60	50	39	29	19	12	5	0	0	0	0
740	750	62	51	41	30	20	13	6	0	0	0	0
750	760	63	53	42	32	21	14	7	0	0	0	0
760	770	65	54	44	33	23	15	8	1	0	0	0
770	780	66	56	45	35	24	16	9	2	0	0	0
780	790	68	57	47	36	26	17	10	3	0	0	0
790	800	69	59	48	38	27	18	11	4	0	0	0
800	810	71	60	50	39	29	19	12	5	0	0	0
810	820	72	62	51	41	30	20	13	6	0	0	0
820	830	74	63	53	42	32	21	14	7	0	0	0
830	840	75	65	54	44	33	23	15	8	1	0	0
840	850	77	66	56	45	35	24	16	9	2	0	0
850	860	78	68	57	47	36	26	17	10	3	0	0
860	870	80	69	59	48	38	27	18	11	4	0	0
870	880	81	71	60	50	39	29	19	12	5	0	0
880	890	83	72	62	51	41	30	20	13	6	0	0
890	900	84	74	63	53	42	32	21	14	7	0	0
900	910	86	75	65	54	44	33	23	15	8	1	0
910	920	87	77	66	56	45	35	24	16	9	2	0
920	930	89	78	68	57	47	36	26	17	10	3	0
930	940	90	80	69	59	48	38	27	18	11	4	0
940	950	92	81	71	60	50	39	29	19	12	5	0
950	960	93	83	72	62	51	41	30	20	13	6	0
960	970	95	84	74	63	53	42	32	21	14	7	0
970	980	96	86	75	65	54	44	33	23	15	8	1
980	990	98	87	77	66	56	45	35	24	16	9	2
990	1000	99	89	78	68	57	47	36	26	17	10	3
1000	1010	101	90	80	69	59	48	38	27	18	11	4
1010	1020	102	92	81	71	60	50	39	29	19	12	5
1020	1030	104	93	83	72	62	51	41	30	20	13	6
1030	1040	105	95	84	74	63	53	42	32	21	14	7
1040	1050	107	96	86	75	65	54	44	33	23	15	8
1050	1060	108	98	87	77	66	56	45	35	24	16	9
1060	1070	110	99	89	78	68	57	47	36	26	17	10
1070	1080	111	101	90	80	69	59	48	38	27	18	11
1080	1090	113	102	92	81	71	60	50	39	29	19	12
1090	1100	114	104	93	83	72	62	51	41	30	20	13
1100	1110	116	105	95	84	74	63	53	42	32	21	14

FIGURE 1-31: (*continued*)

Adapted from Circular E, Employer's Tax Guide. U.S. Department of the Treasury, Internal Revenue Service.

STATE Income Tax

MARRIED

WEEKLY Payroll Period

WAGES		EXEMPTIONS CLAIMED										10 or more
At Least	But Less Than	0	1	2	3	4	5	6	7	8	9	
		TAX TO BE WITHHELD										
$0	$100	$0.00										
100	105	0.00										
105	110	0.00										
110	115	0.00	$0.00									
115	120	0.00	0.00									
120	125	0.00	0.00									
125	130	0.00	0.00									
130	135	0.00	0.00	$0.00								
135	140	0.00	0.00	0.00								
140	145	0.00	0.00	0.00								
145	150	0.20	0.00	0.00								
150	160	0.50	0.00	0.00	$0.00							
160	170	0.90	0.10	0.00	0.00							
170	180	1.30	0.50	0.00	0.00	$0.00						
180	190	1.70	0.90	0.10	0.00	0.00						
190	200	2.10	1.30	0.50	0.00	0.00	$0.00					
200	210	2.50	1.70	0.90	0.10	0.00	0.00					
210	220	2.90	2.10	1.30	0.50	0.00	0.00	$0.00				
220	230	3.30	2.50	1.70	0.90	0.20	0.00	0.00				
230	240	3.70	2.90	2.10	1.30	0.60	0.00	0.00	$0.00			
240	250	4.10	3.30	2.50	1.70	1.00	0.20	0.00	0.00	$0.00		
250	260	4.50	3.70	2.90	2.10	1.40	0.60	0.00	0.00	0.00		
260	270	4.90	4.10	3.30	2.50	1.80	1.00	0.20	0.00	0.00	$0.00	
270	280	5.30	4.50	3.70	2.90	2.20	1.40	0.60	0.00	0.00	0.00	
280	290	5.70	4.90	4.10	3.30	2.60	1.80	1.00	0.30	0.00	0.00	$0.00
290	300	6.10	5.30	4.50	3.70	3.00	2.20	1.40	0.70	0.00	0.00	0.00
300	310	6.50	5.70	4.90	4.10	3.40	2.60	1.80	1.10	0.30	0.00	0.00
310	320	6.90	6.10	5.30	4.50	3.80	3.00	2.20	1.50	0.70	0.00	0.00
320	330	7.40	6.50	5.70	4.90	4.20	3.40	2.60	1.90	1.10	0.30	0.00
330	340	7.80	7.00	6.10	5.30	4.60	3.80	3.00	2.30	1.50	0.70	0.00
340	350	8.30	7.40	6.60	5.70	5.00	4.20	3.40	2.70	1.90	1.10	0.40
350	360	8.70	7.90	7.00	6.10	5.40	4.60	3.80	3.10	2.30	1.50	0.80
360	370	9.30	8.30	7.50	6.60	5.80	5.00	4.20	3.50	2.70	1.90	1.20
370	380	9.80	8.80	7.90	7.00	6.20	5.40	4.60	3.90	3.10	2.30	1.60
380	390	10.30	9.30	8.40	7.50	6.60	5.80	5.00	4.30	3.50	2.70	2.00
390	400	10.80	9.80	8.80	7.90	7.10	6.20	5.40	4.70	3.90	3.10	2.40
400	410	11.40	10.40	9.30	8.40	7.50	6.70	5.80	5.10	4.30	3.50	2.80

FIGURE 1-32: Sample Page from *State Withholding Tax Table and Methods–NY State:* Married Taxpayers, Weekly Payroll Period.

410	420	12.00	10.90	9.90	8.90	8.00	7.10	6.20	5.50	4.70	3.90	3.20
420	430	12.06	11.50	10.40	9.40	8.40	7.60	6.70	5.90	5.10	4.30	3.60
430	440	13.20	12.10	10.90	9.90	8.90	8.00	7.10	6.30	5.50	4.70	4.00
440	450	13.80	12.70	11.50	10.40	9.40	8.50	7.60	6.70	5.90	5.10	4.40
450	460	14.40	13.20	12.10	11.00	9.90	8.90	8.00	7.20	6.30	5.50	4.80
460	470	15.00	13.80	12.70	11.60	10.50	9.50	8.50	7.60	6.80	5.90	5.20
470	480	15.60	14.40	13.30	12.20	11.00	10.00	9.00	8.10	7.20	6.30	5.60
480	490	16.20	15.00	13.90	12.70	11.60	10.50	9.50	8.50	7.70	6.80	6.00
490	500	16.70	15.60	14.50	13.30	12.20	11.10	10.00	9.00	8.10	7.20	6.40
500	510	17.30	16.20	15.10	13.90	12.80	11.70	10.60	9.50	8.60	7.70	6.80
510	520	17.90	16.80	15.70	14.50	13.40	12.20	11.10	10.10	9.10	8.10	7.30
520	530	18.50	17.40	16.20	15.10	14.00	12.80	11.70	10.60	9.60	8.60	7.70
530	540	19.20	18.00	16.80	15.70	14.60	13.40	12.30	11.20	10.10	9.10	8.20
540	550	19.90	18.60	17.40	16.30	15.20	14.00	12.90	11.80	10.60	9.60	8.60
550	560	20.50	19.20	18.00	16.90	15.70	14.60	13.50	12.30	11.20	10.10	9.10
560	570	21.20	19.90	18.60	17.50	16.30	15.20	14.10	12.90	11.80	10.70	9.70
570	580	21.90	20.60	19.30	18.10	16.90	15.80	14.70	13.50	12.40	11.30	10.20
580	590	22.60	21.30	20.00	18.60	17.50	16.40	15.20	14.10	13.00	11.80	10.70
590	600	23.30	22.00	20.60	19.30	18.10	17.00	15.80	14.70	13.60	12.40	11.30
600	610	24.00	22.60	21.30	20.00	18.70	17.60	16.40	15.30	14.20	13.00	11.90
610	620	24.60	23.30	22.00	20.70	19.40	18.10	17.00	15.90	14.70	13.60	12.50
620	630	25.30	24.00	22.70	21.40	20.10	18.70	17.60	16.50	15.30	14.20	13.10
630	640	26.00	24.70	23.40	22.10	20.70	19.40	18.20	17.10	15.90	14.80	13.70
640	650	26.70	25.40	24.10	22.70	21.40	20.10	18.80	17.70	16.50	15.40	14.20

Adapted from State Withholding Tax Table and Methods–NY State. The New York State Department of Taxation and Finance.

FIGURE 1-32: (*continued*)

Examine the following calculations, which combine the figures already calculated. The employee makes a gross wage of $600.00 weekly and has two withholding allowances:

$600.00	Gross pay
20.00	Federal withholding
21.30	State withholding
37.20	Social Security
8.70	Medicare
$512.80	Net payroll

To write a check for net payroll, place the check register and checks on the pegboard, as already demonstrated and record the amount of payroll on the check register under the proper headings. Include the amounts for the federal, state, Social Security, Medicare, and Gross as shown in **Figure 1-33**.

Put the gross amount in the appropriate column on the check register, and put the total deductions in the discount column on the check register.

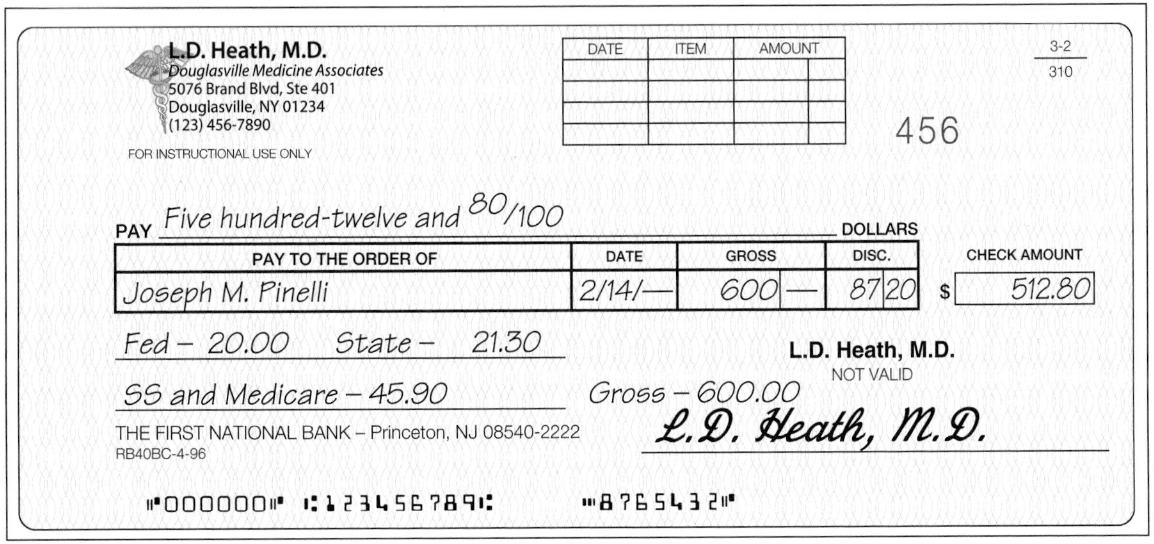

L.D. Heath, M.D.
Douglasville Medicine Associates
5076 Brand Blvd, Ste 401
Douglasville, NY 01234
(123) 456-7890

FOR INSTRUCTIONAL USE ONLY

456

3-2
310

PAY _Five hundred-twelve and 80/100_

PAY TO THE ORDER OF _Joseph M. Pinelli_

DATE	ITEM	AMOUNT

DOLLARS

Fed – 20.00   State – 21.30
SS and Medicare – 45.90

Gross – 600.00

DATE	GROSS	DISC.
2/14/–	600 ––	87 20

CHECK AMOUNT
$ 512.80

L.D. Heath, M.D.
NOT VALID

L.D. Heath, M.D.

THE FIRST NATIONAL BANK – Princeton, NJ 08540-2222
RB40BC-4-96

⑈000000⑈ ⑆123456789⑆ ⑈876543 21⑈

CHECK REGISTER

RECORD OF CHECKS DRAWN ON _____ / _____ PAGE NO.
MONTH OF _February_

LINE NO.	MEMO	PAID TO	DATE	GROSS AMOUNT	DISCOUNT	AMOUNT OF CHECK	CHECK NO	(MEMO) BANK BALANCE			(MEMO) BANK DEPOSIT	
						BALANCE FORWARD		2,769 94			DATE	AMOUNT
1		Joseph M. Pinelli	2/14/–	600 ––	87 20	512 80	456	2,257 14			1	
2											2	
3											3	
4											4	

MONTH OF _February_

	12 Federal Withholding	13 State Withholding	14 SS & Medicare	15 Net Payroll
	20 ––	21 30	45 90	512 80

© Cengage Learning 2013

FIGURE 1-33: Net Payroll Check; Entries in Check Register.

PROCEDURE 11: INSURANCE COVERAGE

Many patients are confused about which type of insurance plan will best meet their needs. Options include many diverse insurance plans, and the medical office professional needs to be aware of the different types of insurance coverage available to patients.

Traditional Insurance Plans and Managed Care Organizations

A traditional plan, also known as an indemnity plan, offers the patient greater flexibility and decision making, provides access to any provider the patient wishes to see, and allows the patient to choose any hospital or specialist for care. This greater freedom in medical care comes with a price. Traditional insurances use a fee-for-service pay schedule, which consists of usual, reasonable, and customary charges. Usual refers to the fee typically charged by a physician for a certain procedure; Reasonable refers to the midrange of fees charged for a particular service; and Customary refers to the average charge for a specific procedure by all physicians practicing the same specialty in a defined geographic and socioeconomic area. A traditional plan usually has a higher deductible, a co-pay, and sometimes a co-insurance where the patient might pay 20% of the medical expense**s** up to a specific limit. Managed Care Organizations (MCO) list the physicians from which the patient may select and determines if and who a patient can see if a specialist is needed. If a patient sees a specialist without the MCO's approval, the patient may have to pay a larger portion of the bill or the entire expense. MCOs also require patients to pay co-pays at the time of service and may also have a deductible, but the main advantage of a managed care system is lower premiums, making health care more affordable for many people. Physicians who join a MCO sign a contract stating that they will accept the payment allowed by the MCO. The difference between what the physician charged and what the MCO paid must be written off and not charged to the patient. An example of a traditional insurance plan would be Blue Cross/ Blue Shield (BC/BC), which is available in all 50 states and may be for-profit or nonprofit. If a physician is participating in the traditional insurance plan, the payment received from the insurance carrier must be accepted as payment and any difference will be written off just as it is in the MCO plans. However, if a patient chooses to see a physician who is not participating with the traditional insurance, the patient will have to pay the difference between the charge and the insurance payment. For some patients, spending more money for a traditional insurance plan may be worth the freedom to choose a physician of choice and having more decision making in their care.

The term *Managed Care Organization (MCO)* is a broad term that describes a system of health care that provides health insurance while controlling costs. There are different types of MCOs. A few examples of MCOs include **health maintenance organizations (HMOs)** and **preferred provider organizations (PPOs).**

The managed care system works by providing comprehensive medical care to members through participating physicians, other health care professionals, and hospitals for a prepaid annual or monthly fee. Ideally, members should be able to have all their medical needs met through the managed care system. When a patient enrolls in an HMO, he or she chooses a PCP from the list of participating physicians who will be responsible for coordinating and managing the patient's care. The PCP has joined the HMO and has signed a contract to accept the prearranged fee schedule payments of the HMO. If the patient needs to be seen by a specialist, the PCP will make a referral for the patient to see a specialist, usually one who is a member of the HMO. Patients who are members of an HMO are given the option of different plans that offer a variety of out-of-pocket expenses and can choose a plan that best fits their budget and the needs of their family.

A PPO is similar to an HMO but it consists of a group of local physicians who joined together and contracted with an MCO to provide care to patients at an agreed-on fee. The patients usually pay a co-pay at the time of visit, like patients enrolled in an HMO, and may need a referral from the PCP to see a specialist. Managed care programs enforce restrictions that traditional health insurance plans do not. For example, nearly all managed care organizations monitor the medical care given to members. Complete, accurate records are important for an MCO's qualification status, as well as for the evaluation of its affiliated hospitals, physicians, and other participating health care professionals. The medical office professional has the responsibility to keep accurate, well-documented medical records.

The HMO-participating physicians are reimbursed in various manners. Some HMOs pay fee-for service, with the HMO deciding on the usual, reasonable, and customary charge. **Capitation** is another way to reimburse the physician. Capitation uses the number of enrolled patients to determine the amount of payment to the physician. A prepaid, fixed, per capita amount is paid for each patient served each month, without consideration to the actual amount of service provided to each patient. Even if the patient is not seen during any given month, the physician is still paid for that patient. This type of reimbursement depends on having many patients enrolled in this specific plan in order to balance out the cost of the medical care. Recording payment from HMOs using capitation payment has created some confusion among offices. The medical office professional needs to become familiar with the procedure used by their office for recording the payment received by this method. If a patient is seen during the month, some offices put through the charge as usual, accept the co-pay, and leave the balance on the ledger card. When the bulk payment check arrives, the capitation amount is applied in the payment column and the difference between the payment and charge is put in the adjustment column, making the balance zero (**see Figures 1-34 and 1-35**). If no services are rendered during a month, some offices enter a charge equal to the amount of payment from the HMO on the ledger card, acknowledging the capitation payment. Be aware that each office has its own procedure for handling these payments, and this simulation has chosen to show only two of the various ways payments can be handled.

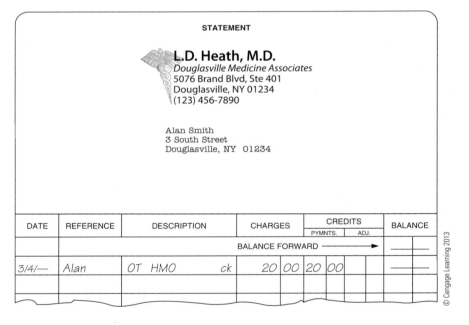

FIGURE 1-34: First Example of a Capitation Payment Method.

FIGURE 1-35: Second Example of a Capitation Payment Method.

Government Funded Insurance

Federal and state governments offer a number of health insurance benefit plans. The medical office professional needs to have a basic understanding of these insurances in order to comply with the state and federal laws when submitting insurance claims.

Medicare   Medicare is a federal insurance program for people over the age of 65 years and older and for individuals with disabilities and end-stage renal disease. Medicare is divided into four parts:

- **Part A Medicare** helps cover hospital expenses, skilled nursing facilities, home health care, and hospice care. Most people do not pay premiums due to paying into the system with payroll taxes while working. Part A Medicare has a substantial deductible, $1,100 for 2010, and a co-insurance amount for hospital stays lasting longer than 60 days.

- **Part B Medicare** helps pay for visits to the physician and other outpatient services such as laboratory tests, radiology services, ambulance service, and durable medical equipment such as wheelchairs, walkers, and commodes but usually does not cover prescription drugs. The patient must pay a monthly premium, which is based on income, and also pay an annual deductible, $155.00 for 2010, before medical outpatient services are paid. Medicare pays 80% of the allowed charge and the patient is responsible for the remaining 20%. Many patients opt for a secondary insurance, referred to as **Medigap** insurance, because it is designed to fill the gap of expenses that Medicare does not cover such as the deductible and the 20% of the expenses. Medicare uses a fee schedule to determine the **resource-based relative value units (RBRVUs),** which are used to set the payments for Part B. A national value for each service performed based on the technical skills required, the amount of time needed to perform the service, malpractice and office overhead expenses, salaries for employees, supplies needed for the procedures, and the costs of living variations in the different geographical area where the physician practices are considered when determining the allowed amount for the services.

- **Part C Medicare** plans, also known as Medicare Advantage plans, are alternate plans to the original Medicare plan and are offered by approved private insurance carriers. Advantage plans combine Part A and Part B Medicare plus many services not covered by the original Parts A and B so patients do not need to purchase supplemental (secondary) insurance. For example, Advantage plans may cover health and wellness programs such as vision and hearing, and most include prescription drug coverage. An advantage plan is a lower-cost alternative to the original Medicare Plan even with the secondary or Medigap insurance plans purchased with the original Medicare Parts A and B. A number of Medicare Advantage plans for selection may be purchased through a regional plan by anyone qualified to receive Medicare benefits when the plan is accepting new members.

- **Part D Medicare** is the prescription drug plan. Part D plans cover both brand-name and generic prescription drugs at participating pharmacies and is beneficial for individuals who have high drug costs or may have unexpected drugs bills in the future. A number of drug plans are available and the individual must consider cost, and the drugs covered since Part D plans are not all alike. It is important for individuals to carefully select the plan that is right for them and will cover the drugs that the individual needs either for treatment or for preventative measures. In most plans, the patient pays a deductible, which includes drug expenses up to $310. Then the patient and the drug plan contribute their portions including the deductible until a combined $2,840 has been reached. The next phase of payment, called the "**donut hole,**" is a coverage gap previously requiring the patient to pay 100% of drug expenses up to a certain amount. Due to the Patient Protection and Affordable Care Act of 2010, a law that reduced the amount of money a patient had to pay while in the "donut hole," patients in 2011 will be given a 50% discount on prescription drugs. According to the law, by 2020, effective changes will be to decrease the 50% discount in the "donut hole" to 25%. After the patient reaches the required amount for the "donut hole," the plan will pay most of the drug expenses and the patient will pay only a small co-pay.

Medicaid   Medicaid insurance, created in 1965 as Title XIX, is a jointly sponsored federal and state health program administered by state governments, which is designed to help low-income and disabled individuals. Each state develops its own rules and regulations concerning eligibility and benefit packages such as the type of benefits and the amount of payments made to the individual. Because Medicaid is based on need, income and other financial assets must be made available. Federal law states that a benefit package includes inpatient hospital care, outpatient services, physician services, diagnostic procedures such as laboratory and radiology, skilled nursing facilities, and home care. Some states may add other services to the medical package benefits such as dental and prescription coverage. Some states require a small co-pay at the time of service. A physician participating with Medicaid follows the same rules and regulations regarding payments of services given. The difference between the physician's charge for a service and the payment received from Medicaid will be written off as an adjustment and the patient will not be billed. If the patient has other insurances, Medicaid will always be the last insurer and not the primary insurer.

Tricare   **Tricare**, formerly known as **CHAMPUS** (Civilian Health and Medical Program of the Uniformed Services), is the health care program offered by the Department of Defense for members of uniformed services both active and retired, their families, and survivors. Tricare is a major component of the military health system, which provides a patient with Army, Navy, and Air Force military health care resources supplemented with civilian health care resources. Tricare offers three main health care choices: Tricare Prime, Tricare Extra, and Tricare Standard. Eligible individuals may select from the plan that best meets their needs and the needs of their family members. Tricare standard, the original CHAMPUS, is one of the insurance options available to retirees and their dependants based on a fee-for-service plan and usually requires a higher out-of-pocket cost. Tricare Extra is another plan available to retirees and their dependants. A person enrolled in this plan selects a physician from a "preferred" or participating list of physicians who agree to the payments allowed by the program. The patient is not required to see a Tricare-preferred physician but there is less out-of-pocket expense if he or she sees a physician in the network. Tricare Prime, similar to an HMO, is the plan in which active military personnel are automatically enrolled, although retirees and their dependants may also chose to enroll in this plan. Most care is provided through military hospitals and other military facilities. This plan offers the greatest coverage of the three main Tricare plans, especially for preventive and primary care services. Active military personnel do not pay a yearly enrollment fee because participation in this plan is required. Other beneficiaries must enroll annually for this plan.

Each patient coming to the medical office who has Tricare will have a membership card containing the information about services covered and claim payment regulations. Tricare can be a primary or secondary insurance depending of the type of plan, and there may be deductibles and co-pay.

Workers' Compensation **Workers' Compensation** is a form of medical benefits and wage replacement required by law for an employee injured on the job or due to an illness related to the job. Insurance claims for a patient with a Workers' Compensation claim are not sent to the patient's primary insurance but rather to the patient's employer's Workers' Compensation insurance provider, who will take over the claim process. The medical office does not send the patient a bill. The physician may have the responsibility to send requested reports but is not involved in the billing process after the initial bill is sent to the employer's Workers' Compensation insurance. Each state has its own Workers' Compensation laws.

Responsibilities of the Medical Office Professional

The medical office professional working in an outpatient medical facility has the responsibility to verify the insurance information of each patient being treated, regardless of the type of insurance. When scheduling an appointment, you should remind each patient to bring his or her insurance card to the appointment. Make a copy of both sides of the patient's insurance card and keep this information on file in the patient's medical record. Always file the claim to the primary insurance carrier first when filing claims for patients with more than one insurance carrier—Tricare and Medicaid are billed after private insurance for patients with both types of coverage. If an injury was caused by an accident and is covered by automobile or homeowner's insurance, this insurance becomes the primary carrier. If a patient is requesting an appointment due to an injury, ask if the injury is a Workers' Compensation case so that the claim will not be sent to the patient's primary insurance.

Although identification cards may vary, most cards will contain similar information. The Medicare ID card (as shown in **Figure 1-36**) lists the patient's name, the Medicare claim number, gender, effective date of the insurance coverage, the parts of Medicare the patient is entitled to such as Part A and Part B, and the patient's signature. Information about the insurance carrier is listed on the back of the card such as where to mail claims, the number to call for questions, the mailing address for the claim if needed, and many times the payer code for electronic submission of claims. Many offices have a **point-of-service (POS) device (Figure 1-37)**, which allows direct communication between a medical office and the insurance carrier's computer system to check the insurance eligibility of a patient, to enter data such as referral information, and for authorization verification. The patient's ID card is swiped through the machine, which is similar to a credit card machine, or the patient's ID number is entered on the keypad. An immediate response from the plan's computer is received in the office verifying the eligibility of the patient's insurance or other information requested.

When working with patient insurances, always file with Medicare before filing with a supplemental carrier. If preparing a paper copy of the insurance claim form,

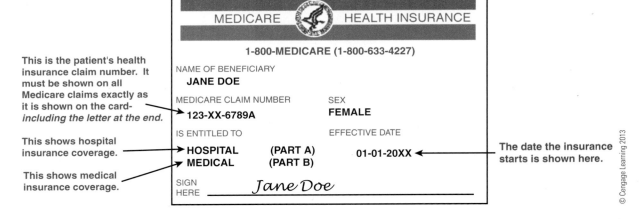

FIGURE 1-36: Medicare Health Insurance Card.

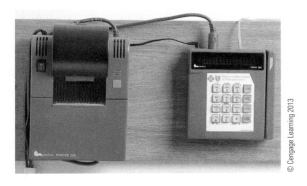

FIGURE 1-37: Point-of-Service (POS) device.

include a copy of the EOB (Explanation of Benefits) from Medicare when filing with the supplemental carrier. Medicaid, or medical assistance patients must be currently authorized. Medicaid claims should be filed after all other health insurance. Medicaid rules and regulations are constantly being updated, and medical office professionals must keep up with the latest changes. Some states allow physicians to charge Medicaid patients a small co-payment for health care services. This charge may or may not be required by your physician-employer; in some states, physicians cannot collect any money from Medicaid patients so any amount not allowed and not paid will need to be written off as an adjustment. For example: A claim was submitted to Medicaid for $177.00 and Medicaid paid $90.50. The remaining balance of $86.50 would have to be written off as an adjustment, because the physician is not allowed to bill the patient for the remaining amount of the bill.

An insurance file should be set up for quick reference to hold information about all insurance carriers used by the office. To avoid delays in reimbursement, obtain all insurance and payment information from the patient as early as possible. Most insurance carriers have between a 90- and a 120-day period in which the office can submit a claim to be paid. Ask new patients about insurance coverage when they make their appointments to be sure your facility is participating in the patient's insurance, requesting that the insurance card be brought to the appointment to be photocopied.

PROCEDURE 12: INSURANCE CODING

The CMS-1500 insurance claim form **(see Figure 1-38)** is used to process insurance claims, adding all the necessary information for accurate processing. Two main coding systems are used when completing insurance claims. The **International Classification-Clinical Modification (ICD-CM)** is used in coding patient diagnoses and the **Current Procedural Terminology (CPT)** is used in coding patient procedures and services.

ICD-9-CM and ICD-10-CM Diagnostic Codes

The ICD is a diagnosis classification system that translates a diagnosis into a number system to allow systematic tracking, recording, analysis, and interpretation of the various disease conditions and health management issues from all over the world. With a numbered system, mortality and morbidity rates can be analyzed and compared with different countries around the world. The United States has modified the ICD, thus renaming it ICD-CM, which stands for Clinical Modification. The "9"in the ICD-9-CM is the edition that the modification was released for use and is updated at intervals. The **Centers for Medicare and Medicaid Services (CMS)**, the financing department previously known as the Health Care Financing Administration (HCFA), developed the diagnostic coding system based on the ICD for use by all health providers.

1500

HEALTH INSURANCE CLAIM FORM
APPROVED BY NATIONAL UNIFORM CLAIM COMMITTEE 08/05

PICA				PICA

1. MEDICARE (Medicare #) MEDICAID (Medicaid #) TRICARE CHAMPUS (Sponsor's SSN) CHAMPVA (Member ID#) GROUP HEALTH PLAN (SSN or ID) FECA BLK LUNG (SSN) OTHER (ID) | 1a. INSURED'S I.D. NUMBER (For Program in Item 1)

2. PATIENT'S NAME (Last Name, First Name, Middle Initial) | 3. PATIENT'S BIRTH DATE MM DD YY SEX M F | 4. INSURED'S NAME (Last Name, First Name, Middle Initial)

5. PATIENT'S ADDRESS (No., Street) | 6. PATIENT RELATIONSHIP TO INSURED Self Spouse Child Other | 7. INSURED'S ADDRESS (No., Street)

CITY STATE | 8. PATIENT STATUS Single Married Other | CITY STATE

ZIP CODE TELEPHONE (Include Area Code) ( ) | Employed Full-Time Student Part-Time Student | ZIP CODE TELEPHONE (Include Area Code) ( )

9. OTHER INSURED'S NAME (Last Name, First Name, Middle Initial) | 10. IS PATIENT'S CONDITION RELATED TO: | 11. INSURED'S POLICY GROUP OR FECA NUMBER

a. OTHER INSURED'S POLICY OR GROUP NUMBER | a. EMPLOYMENT? (Current or Previous) YES NO | a. INSURED'S DATE OF BIRTH MM DD YY SEX M F

b. OTHER INSURED'S DATE OF BIRTH MM DD YY SEX M F | b. AUTO ACCIDENT? PLACE (State) YES NO | b. EMPLOYER'S NAME OR SCHOOL NAME

c. EMPLOYER'S NAME OR SCHOOL NAME | c. OTHER ACCIDENT? YES NO | c. INSURANCE PLAN NAME OR PROGRAM NAME

d. INSURANCE PLAN NAME OR PROGRAM NAME | 10d. RESERVED FOR LOCAL USE | d. IS THERE ANOTHER HEALTH BENEFIT PLAN? YES NO If yes, return to and complete item 9 a-d.

READ BACK OF FORM BEFORE COMPLETING & SIGNING THIS FORM.
12. PATIENT'S OR AUTHORIZED PERSON'S SIGNATURE I authorize the release of any medical or other information necessary to process this claim. I also request payment of government benefits either to myself or to the party who accepts assignment below.

SIGNED _____ DATE _____

13. INSURED'S OR AUTHORIZED PERSON'S SIGNATURE I authorize payment of medical benefits to the undersigned physician or supplier for services described below.

SIGNED _____

14. DATE OF CURRENT: MM DD YY ILLNESS (First symptom) OR INJURY (Accident) OR PREGNANCY(LMP) | 15. IF PATIENT HAS HAD SAME OR SIMILAR ILLNESS. GIVE FIRST DATE MM DD YY | 16. DATES PATIENT UNABLE TO WORK IN CURRENT OCCUPATION FROM MM DD YY TO MM DD YY

17. NAME OF REFERRING PROVIDER OR OTHER SOURCE 17a. 17b. NPI | 18. HOSPITALIZATION DATES RELATED TO CURRENT SERVICES FROM MM DD YY TO MM DD YY

19. RESERVED FOR LOCAL USE | 20. OUTSIDE LAB? YES NO $ CHARGES

21. DIAGNOSIS OR NATURE OF ILLNESS OR INJURY (Relate Items 1, 2, 3 or 4 to Item 24E by Line)
1. ____ . ____   3. ____ . ____
2. ____ . ____   4. ____ . ____ | 22. MEDICAID RESUBMISSION CODE ORIGINAL REF. NO.
23. PRIOR AUTHORIZATION NUMBER

24. A. DATE(S) OF SERVICE From MM DD YY To MM DD YY	B. PLACE OF SERVICE	C. EMG	D. PROCEDURES, SERVICES, OR SUPPLIES (Explain Unusual Circumstances) CPT/HCPCS	MODIFIER	E. DIAGNOSIS POINTER	F. $ CHARGES	G. DAYS OR UNITS	H. EPSDT Family Plan	I. ID. QUAL.	J. RENDERING PROVIDER ID. #
1										NPI
2										NPI
3										NPI
4										NPI
5										NPI
6										NPI

25. FEDERAL TAX I.D. NUMBER SSN EIN | 26. PATIENT'S ACCOUNT NO. | 27. ACCEPT ASSIGNMENT? (For govt. claims, see back) YES NO | 28. TOTAL CHARGE $ | 29. AMOUNT PAID $ | 30. BALANCE DUE $

31. SIGNATURE OF PHYSICIAN OR SUPPLIER INCLUDING DEGREES OR CREDENTIALS (I certify that the statements on the reverse apply to this bill and are made a part thereof.)
SIGNED _____ DATE _____ | 32. SERVICE FACILITY LOCATION INFORMATION a. NPI b. | 33. BILLING PROVIDER INFO & PH # ( ) a. NPI b.

NUCC Instruction Manual available at: www.nucc.org APPROVED OMB-0938-0999 FORM CMS-1500 (08/05)

CARRIER
PATIENT AND INSURED INFORMATION
PHYSICIAN OR SUPPLIER INFORMATION

FIGURE 1-38: CMS-1500 Claim Form (Front and Back).

BECAUSE THIS FORM IS USED BY VARIOUS GOVERNMENT AND PRIVATE HEALTH PROGRAMS, SEE SEPARATE INSTRUCTIONS ISSUED BY APPLICABLE PROGRAMS.

NOTICE: Any person who knowingly files a statement of claim containing any misrepresentation or any false, incomplete or misleading information may be guilty of a criminal act punishable under law and may be subject to civil penalties.

REFERS TO GOVERNMENT PROGRAMS ONLY

MEDICARE AND CHAMPUS PAYMENTS: A patient's signature requests that payment be made and authorizes release of any information necessary to process the claim and certifies that the information provided in Blocks 1 through 12 is true, accurate and complete. In the case of a Medicare claim, the patient's signature authorizes any entity to release to Medicare medical and nonmedical information, including employment status, and whether the person has employer group health insurance, liability, no-fault, worker's compensation or other insurance which is responsible to pay for the services for which the Medicare claim is made. See 42 CFR 411.24(a). If item 9 is completed, the patient's signature authorizes release of the information to the health plan or agency shown. In Medicare assigned or CHAMPUS participation cases, the physician agrees to accept the charge determination of the Medicare carrier or CHAMPUS fiscal intermediary as the full charge, and the patient is responsible only for the deductible, coinsurance and noncovered services. Coinsurance and the deductible are based upon the charge determination of the Medicare carrier or CHAMPUS fiscal intermediary if this is less than the charge submitted. CHAMPUS is not a health insurance program but makes payment for health benefits provided through certain affiliations with the Uniformed Services. Information on the patient's sponsor should be provided in those items captioned in "Insured"; i.e., items 1a, 4, 6, 7, 9, and 11.

BLACK LUNG AND FECA CLAIMS

The provider agrees to accept the amount paid by the Government as payment in full. See Black Lung and FECA instructions regarding required procedure and diagnosis coding systems.

SIGNATURE OF PHYSICIAN OR SUPPLIER (MEDICARE, CHAMPUS, FECA AND BLACK LUNG)

I certify that the services shown on this form were medically indicated and necessary for the health of the patient and were personally furnished by me or were furnished incident to my professional service by my employee under my immediate personal supervision, except as otherwise expressly permitted by Medicare or CHAMPUS regulations.

For services to be considered as "incident" to a physician's professional service, 1) they must be rendered under the physician's immediate personal supervision by his/her employee, 2) they must be an integral, although incidental part of a covered physician's service, 3) they must be of kinds commonly furnished in physician's offices, and 4) the services of nonphysicians must be included on the physician's bills.

For CHAMPUS claims, I further certify that I (or any employee) who rendered services am not an active duty member of the Uniformed Services or a civilian employee of the United States Government or a contract employee of the United States Government, either civilian or military (refer to 5 USC 5536). For Black-Lung claims, I further certify that the services performed were for a Black Lung-related disorder.

No Part B Medicare benefits may be paid unless this form is received as required by existing law and regulations (42 CFR 424.32).

NOTICE: Any one who misrepresents or falsifies essential information to receive payment from Federal funds requested by this form may upon conviction be subject to fine and imprisonment under applicable Federal laws.

NOTICE TO PATIENT ABOUT THE COLLECTION AND USE OF MEDICARE, CHAMPUS, FECA, AND BLACK LUNG INFORMATION
(PRIVACY ACT STATEMENT)

We are authorized by HCFA, CHAMPUS and OWCP to ask you for information needed in the administration of the Medicare, CHAMPUS, FECA, and Black Lung programs. Authority to collect information is in section 205(a), 1862, 1872 and 1874 of the Social Security Act as amended, 42 CFR 411.24(a) and 424.5(a) (6), and 44 USC 3101;41 CFR 101 et seq and 10 USC 1079 and 1086; 5 USC 8101 et seq; and 30 USC 901 et seq; 38 USC 613; E.O. 9397.

The information we obtain to complete claims under these programs is used to identify you and to determine your eligibility. It is also used to decide if the services and supplies you received are covered by these programs and to insure that proper payment is made.

The information may also be given to other providers of services, carriers, intermediaries, medical review boards, health plans, and other organizations or Federal agencies, for the effective administration of Federal provisions that require other third parties payers to pay primary to Federal program, and as otherwise necessary to administer these programs. For example, it may be necessary to disclose information about the benefits you have used to a hospital or doctor. Additional disclosures are made through routine uses for information contained in systems of records.

FOR MEDICARE CLAIMS: See the notice modifying system No. 09-70-0501, titled, 'Carrier Medicare Claims Record,' published in the Federal Register, Vol. 55 No. 177, page 37549, Wed. Sept. 12, 1990, or as updated and republished.

FOR OWCP CLAIMS: Department of Labor, Privacy Act of 1974, "Republication of Notice of Systems of Records," Federal Register Vol. 55 No. 40, Wed Feb. 28, 1990, See ESA-5, ESA-6, ESA-12, ESA-13, ESA-30, or as updated and republished.

FOR CHAMPUS CLAIMS: PRINCIPLE PURPOSE(S): To evaluate eligibility for medical care provided by civilian sources and to issue payment upon establishment of eligibility and determination that the services/supplies received are authorized by law.

ROUTINE USE(S): Information from claims and related documents may be given to the Dept. of Veterans Affairs, the Dept. of Health and Human Services and/or the Dept. of Transportation consistent with their statutory administrative responsibilities under CHAMPUS/CHAMPVA; to the Dept. of Justice for representation of the Secretary of Defense in civil actions; to the Internal Revenue Service, private collection agencies, and consumer reporting agencies in connection with recoupment claims; and to Congressional Offices in response to inquiries made at the request of the person to whom a record pertains. Appropriate disclosures may be made to other federal, state, local, foreign government agencies, private business entities, and individual providers of care, on matters relating to entitlement, claims adjudication, fraud, program abuse, utilization review, quality assurance, peer review, program integrity, third-party liability, coordination of benefits, and civil and criminal litigation related to the operation of CHAMPUS.

DISCLOSURES: Voluntary; however, failure to provide information will result in delay in payment or may result in denial of claim. With the one exception discussed below, there are no penalties under these programs for refusing to supply information. However, failure to furnish information regarding the medical services rendered or the amount charged would prevent payment of claims under these programs. Failure to furnish any other information, such as name or claim number, would delay payment of the claim. Failure to provide medical information under FECA could be deemed an obstruction.

It is mandatory that you tell us if you know that another party is responsible for paying for your treatment. Section 1128B of the Social Security Act and 31 USC 3801-3812 provide penalties for withholding this information.

You should be aware that P.L. 100-503, the "Computer Matching and Privacy Protection Act of 1988", permits the government to verify information by way of computer matches.

MEDICAID PAYMENTS (PROVIDER CERTIFICATION)

I hereby agree to keep such records as are necessary to disclose fully the extent of services provided to individuals under the State's Title XIX plan and to furnish information regarding any payments claimed for providing such services as the State Agency or Dept. of Health and Humans Services may request.

I further agree to accept, as payment in full, the amount paid by the Medicaid program for those claims submitted for payment under that program, with the exception of authorized deductible, coinsurance, co-payment or similar cost-sharing charge.

SIGNATURE OF PHYSICIAN (OR SUPPLIER): I certify that the services listed above were medically indicated and necessary to the health of this patient and were personally furnished by me or my employee under my personal direction.

NOTICE: This is to certify that the foregoing information is true, accurate and complete. I understand that payment and satisfaction of this claim will be from Federal and State funds, and that any false claims, statements, or documents, or concealment of a material fact, may be prosecuted under applicable Federal or State laws.

Public reporting burden for this collection of information is estimated to average 15 minutes per response, including time for reviewing instructions, searching existing date sources, gathering and maintaining data needed, and completing and reviewing the collection of information. Send comments regarding this burden estimate or any other aspect of this collection of information, including suggestions for reducing the burden, to HCFA, Office of Financial Management, P.O. Box 26684, Baltimore, MD 21207; and to the Office of Management and Budget, Paperwork Reduction Project (OMB-0938-0008), Washington, D.C. 20503.

FIGURE 1-38: (continued)

Centers for Medicare and Medicaid Services.

HIPAA Code Sets, first used in 1996, became the standard in all health care facilities for reporting diseases, injuries, other health problems such as disease impairments, and causes of injuries and poisonings. Health care providers were required to use ICD-9 when it became the official guidelines for coding and reporting in the 1970s. As the years went on and technology and medical knowledge advanced, ICD-9 no longer met the health information needs of the health care system as it contained outdated terminology and classifications and lacked the details needed for the tracking of data and analysis that needed to be done. As early as the 1990s, it was recognized that the ICD-9 system needed to be updated or replaced, but it took many years before a system could be developed that would provide more accuracy and specificity. The National Center for Health Statistics (NCHS), a division of the **Centers for Disease Control and Prevention (CDC),** developed the clinical modification of ICD-10 with the goal of developing a system that would address the quality of health care, provide more exchange of data between health care providers, and provide a method of tracking public health threats, identifying medical errors, and evaluating resource management. The United States is required to report to the **World Health Organization (WHO)** mortality and morbidity data and any new system developed needed to include a better, more accurate way of reporting and comparing **mortality** and **morbidity** statistics and provide the codes for reporting this information.

One of the main reasons for moving to ICD-10 was the improvement in reporting and overcoming the limitations of ICD-9. When ICD-10 came out in 1992, it had broadened its scope, including areas such as increased ambulatory care services, risk factors in primary care, clinical details, and emergent diseases as well as code changes to mental and behavioral disorders, injuries, poisoning, external causes for mortality and morbidity, and categories for postprocedural disorders. ICD-10 codes also provide better data for evaluating and improving the quality of patient care and provide for more detailed clinical documentation. ICD-10 was designed to be more flexible than ICD-9, more adaptable to changes that occur in health care over time due to advances in medical knowledge and technology, and to provide more details for research. From an economic viewpoint, ICD-10 was designed to be more efficient than ICD-9, resulting in lower costs after the initial setup, fewer claim rejections, and reduced coding errors. Detailed codes would provide better and more accurate data.

The final compliance date for using ICD-10 in the United States is October 1, 2013, when the ICD-9-CM procedure code sets will be replaced with ICD-10-CM, which will be used in all health care facilities reporting physician services and procedures performed on an outpatient hospital service or in other outpatient facilities. "The ICD-10-PCS (Procedural Coding System) will be used by facilities reporting in-patient hospital services only. Current Procedural Terminology (CPT) codes will continue to be used for reporting physician services and procedures performed in hospital outpatient departments and other outpatient facilities" (Zeisset, 2010, p.15). Compliance with ICD-10-CM is important because it is the international standard for reporting and monitoring diseases and mortality making it important for the United States to adopt.

What is the difference between ICD-10 and ICD-9? ICD-10 is different in structure having each code begin with an alphabetic character and containing up to seven characters, unlike the ICD-9, which consists of all numeric digits and a maximum of five digits. The **V codes** (Factors Influencing Health Status and Contact with Health Services) and **E codes** (External Causes of Injury and Poisoning) found as separate entities in ICD-9 are incorporated into the codes for ICD-10, eliminating the need for extra coding steps. ICD-10 has a completely alphanumeric format coding scheme where the first character is a letter, the second character is a numeric digit, and the remaining characters are either a letter or a number. All the letters of the alphabet are used except the letter "U," which is not used unless needed to code a new disease of uncertain origin. The ICD-10-CM has approximately 68,000 codes, whereas the ICD-9-CM has approximately 14,000 codes. The arrangement of the ICD-10 book is similar to that of the ICD-9 book, having an alphabetical and tabular index with the main terms listed in alphabetical order and qualifiers and descriptors indented.

CPT Procedure Codes

Current Procedural Terminology (CPT), 4th edition, is a coding system developed by the American Medical Association (AMA) that lists medical services and procedures performed by physicians and translates them into five digit codes. CPT codes provide a uniform language that can be used to provide accurate communication between patients, physicians, and third-parties for insurance claim processing, research, and development of guidelines for medical care review. CPT was developed in 1966 mainly to standardize procedure terminology among physicians and has been revised three times over the years. As newer editions were developed, CPT became mandated for use in Medicare and Medicaid billing. CPT-4 is now the most widely used coding system for reimbursement among third-party payers. The CPT coding manual is published annually to update new procedures and technology.

Category I codes are primary codes used to describe procedures and are divided into six categories or sections in the CPT manual:

1. Evaluation and Management: 99201–99499
2. Anesthesia: 00100–01999
3. Surgery: 10021–69990
4. Radiology: 70010–79999
5. Pathology and Laboratory: 80047–89398
6. Medicine: 90281–99602

Category II codes are optional and used for informational purposes only. They cannot replace Category I codes. Category II codes may be used to facilitate data collection about quality of care provided and are not used for reimbursement.

Category III codes are used in place of an unlisted code usually for newer technology that has not yet received a code in category I. Reimbursement will be made if the Category III code meets Category I requirements. Reimbursement is made at the determination of the individual insurance carrier.

CPT Modifiers (also referred to as Level I modifiers) are two-digit numbers used to supplement information or adjust descriptions providing extra details about a procedure or service or indicating that it was changed in some way due to specific circumstances. Modifiers are important in the reimbursement process because they help ensure correct reimbursement. They are entered in the same box as the CPT code on the CMS-1500 claim form.

A modifier would be used to indicate, for example, that a bilateral procedure was done or that the procedure was performed by two physicians. If the physician performed a bilateral herniorrhapy, the modifier -50 would indicate that two hernia repair surgeries were performed, one on the right side and one on the left side. The physician would bill for two procedures and get reimbursed for two procedures. If two surgeons were operating on a patient and each one was performing a procedure on a different part of the body, each surgeon would be reimbursed for the surgery he or she performed by using the modifier -62. Another common modifier used is modifier -25, which is used to designate a significant, separately identifiable evaluation and management service by the same physician on the same day of the same procedure or other service. An example of using modifier -25 would be if the patient came in for an office visit and an EKG was performed. The EKG is considered a separate identifiable service performed by the physician on the same day as the office visit, which could have been for evaluation and management of chest pain.

Preparing the Insurance Claim Form

An insurance claim is a request for payment from a health care provider for services furnished to a patient. For years, insurance claims were sent on paper with each insurance carrier having a separate form, but as the insurance industry grew the insurance claims multiplied to a staggering number, along with the numerous calls and resubmission of claims with errors. Although a booming business, the paper claim process became a tremendous burden on the insurance industry, plus a tremendous task for the postal service to handle all the generated mail. Today, most insurance claims are sent electronically using a **clearinghouse**—basically, a service provided for a charge where a company looks over the claims checking for errors. If no errors are present, the clearinghouse sends the claim to the proper insurance carrier following the rules and regulations of HIPAA. If errors are found, the claim is returned to the provider to be fixed before resubmitting it. Using a clearinghouse saves time for both the provider and the insurance carrier because turnaround time for claim processing is faster and more productive due to fewer claims reaching the insurance carrier with errors, which would disqualify the claim from being paid.

The Administrative Simplification Compliance Act (ASCA) of 2003 prohibited the sending of paper claims to Medicare for reimbursement except in limited circumstances. For the providers allowed to send paper claims, an original CMS-1500 form printed in red ink must be used in order to be excepted since the claim is scanned and read by Optical Character Recognition (OCR) technology. Many insurance carriers have set a time limit for claim submission and require that claims be submitted within 90 to 120 days in order to be considered for payment. Physician service claims for Medicare benefits must be submitted within 1 year from the date of service and the patient may not be charged for completion of the insurance form. The CMS-1500, also known as the universal claim form, is accepted by most insurance forms.

In this simulation, you will fill out paper CMS-1500 claim forms for different insurance carriers in order to gain a better understanding of how the information collected at the time of patient registration is used for insurance claim processing. In the second part of the simulation, the information used on the paper claim form will be entered onto the computer.

To complete a universal claim form, do the following:

1. Locate the patient's ledger card.
2. Identify the type of claim by checking the appropriate square in box 1 at the top of the form. If you have checked "Group Health Plan" or "Other," be sure to list the name and address of the insurance company at the top right corner of the form. Obtain this information from the insurer file. Refer to the patient's ledger card to obtain the information needed to complete boxes 1a through 13.
3. Check to be sure the patient's signature is on file and that the HIPAA Privacy Notice has been signed. Mark "signature on file" in box 12 and date the form for the time services were rendered. Be sure to complete box 13 in the same manner, if applicable.
4. Complete boxes 14 and 15, as applicable. In box 14, put the earliest date of service for which the claim is being made, unless the complaint results from an accident or injury. In this case, note the date of the accident or injury. Use box 15 only if the claim is for visits about a continuing condition for which prior claims have been made. In such cases, type the date when the patient first consulted Douglasville Medicine Associates about this condition. For this simulation, ignore boxes 16 through 23.
5. In box 21, add the ICD-CM code(s). The ICD-CM codes you will need for this simulation are found on the inside cover of this book. Each claim form can contain up to four diagnoses. Always check the accuracy of these codes, since insurers will not pay if codes are incorrect. An up-to-date ICD-CM code book should be used since the codes may change and diagnoses need to be coded to the highest level of specificity. For example, if the code book indicates that five digits are needed for the diagnosis, then five digits need to be inserted; less than that would result in denial of the claim and no payment until a correction was made.
6. Fill out box 24 completely. Each letter below refers to a different section of the box.

   A. Put the date of service in both the "From" and "To" boxes.

   B. Refer to the inside front cover for Place of Service Codes.

C. Put the procedure code (CPT code) in the first box. For this simulation put nothing in the Modifier box unless specified. Refer to the inside cover for procedure codes.

D. In this box place the number of the diagnosis (see box 21) to which this procedure refers. For example, if a patient had hypertension and diabetes mellitus, the diagnoses would be listed in box 21—Diagnosis 1: 401.1 and Diagnosis 2: 250.00. In box 24 D, the office visit would be 99213 and column E would record diagnoses 1 and 2 since the patient was seen for both conditions. If a urinalysis (81002) was done to check for glucose in the urine, the diagnosis would be #2 in column E since the urine test was done specifically for diabetes and not for hypertension. With a Medicare claim, the modifier -25 would be used to designate that a separate procedure that did not apply to both diagnoses was done.

F. Note the charges in Box 24 Column F.

G. Fill in a *1* for a one-time (day) service or with the number of days the service was provided (used for daily hospital visits). For this simulation ignore boxes H–K.

7. Box 26 is for physician's use and in this simulation can be left blank.

8. Box 27 is for **accepting assignment**. Accepting assignment means the physician will accept the amount allowed for payment and will not require the patient to pay the difference between the physician's charge and the Medicare amount allowed. Douglasville Medicine Associates accepts assignment for Medicare, Medicaid, HMOs, and most private insurance claims.

9. Box 28 is for the total charge of the claim.

10. Box 29 is filled in if the patient has made a payment.

11. Box 30 is filled in with the amount from Box 28 minus the amount from Box 29.

12. Box 31 does not need to be signed by the physician if the physician has a contract with the insurance carrier.

13. Box 32 is for the facility where the service was performed. If the service was performed at the medical office (POS 11), leave this blank.

14. Box 33 is for the physician's name, address, telephone number, group identification number, and NPI number. In Box 33a, the physician's **National Provider Identification (NPI)** number is entered. The NPI is a unique identification number for health care providers. It is required that all health care providers have an NPI in order to be reimbursed by insurance companies, write prescriptions, or refer patients to other health care providers.

15. The physician no longer has to sign the form in box 31 before you send it.

Recheck the insurance claim to be sure all information needed is written in and all areas are completed (**see Figure 1-39**).

FIGURE 1-39: Completed Claim Form.

SECTION 2

As you work through this simulation, complete all jobs in order. Before you begin work on the simulation, review the Reference Manual (Section 1) and familiarize yourself with what is found in the Section 4 and the Pegboard Forms. Remember to:

- Keep patient ledger cards in alphabetical order for easy access; and
- Legibly complete patient lists, insurance forms, and any information needed on patient ledger cards.

The day sheet for March 4 should be day sheet No. 43.

MARCH				
4	5	6	7	8
Monday	Tuesday	Wednesday	Thursday	Friday

Today you will be working with Dr. Heath. Pull the medical records for today's patients and put them on Dr. Heath's desk in the order of time the patient is to arrive for the appointment. Put the patient list on top of the charts for Dr. Heath's reference. Sort and open the mail, and follow through on any messages left with the answering service.

JOB 1-1

At about 8:50 a.m., Margaret Chandler, a new patient, arrives. Fill in a ledger card using the information Mrs. Chandler provides (use the data from the following box). Mrs. Chandler is concerned about chest pain on exertion. After examining the patient, Dr. Heath orders a stress test to be done today at the hospital. (Because the test is performed outside the office, no procedure code or charge is recorded by your office for the stress test. Charge Mrs. Chandler for an office visit only—Level 2 Office Visit, new patient [99202]; the diagnosis is angina pectoris.) Schedule a return appointment for Thursday, March 7, at 9:15 a.m. for a reexamination (Level 3) of chest pain and discussion of the test results. Mrs. Chandler receives a receipt for her $20 cash payment (refer back to Figure 1-15). Submit the insurance claim for Margaret Chandler. Her signature is on file.

Mrs. Margaret S. Chandler
56 Cold Soil Road
Douglasville, NY 01234
(123) 555-3423

Date of birth: 11/5/1950

Soc. Sec. No.: 388-15-8890

Nearest relative: Timothy P. Chandler (spouse)

Spouse date of birth: 10/9/1949

Spouse Soc. Sec. No.: 043-23-1918

Employer (Margaret): Greenfield, Morgan, and Berman
9100 Academy Road
Douglasville, NY 01234
(123) 555-1900

Insurance: FlexiHealth PPO

ID No.: 388-15-8890

Group No.: 000-2095

Office co-pay: $20

Release: Signature on file, accepts assignment

HIPAA form: Signed and acknowledged; copy given to patient

JOB 1-2

Pamela Cameron, a new patient, arrives for her 10:00 a.m. appointment. Dr. Heath examines Ms. Cameron. Her past history sheet shows that she has been treated for iron-deficiency anemia. At today's visit, she is complaining of pain when urinating and also states that she is tired all the time. Dr. Heath tests a sample of Ms. Cameron's urine and also performs a hematocrit (Hct). Complete the insurance claim for the office visit (Level 2 Office Visit, new patient), Diagnosis 1: Urinary tract infection (599.0), and urine test w/out microscopy (81002); Diagnosis 2: iron-deficiency anemia (280.9), and Hct (85014). Give Ms. Cameron a receipt showing the charge entered on her account and her next appointment on Thursday, March 7, at 10:15 a.m.

Ms. Pamela H. Cameron
453 Woodsville Road
Douglasville, NY 01234
(123) 555-3510

Date of birth: 3/1/74

Soc. Sec. No.: 237-35-2323

Nearest relative: Scott Cameron (spouse)

Employer: Worldwide Travel Agency
300 State Street
Douglasville, NY 01234
(123) 555-8967

Insurance: United Heath Care

ID No.: 237-35-2323

Group No.: 505388
No co-pay, no deductible

Release: Signature on file, accepts assignment

HIPAA form: Signed and copy given to patient

JOB 1-3

Walter Adams, an established patient, arrives for his appointment. He is here today to have his blood pressure checked. Mr. Adams's blood pressure is elevated, so Dr. Heath performs an EKG and will send Mr. Adams to the laboratory to have blood drawn for a cholesterol level (outside laboratory). Mr. Adams requests a superbill, which lists the charges for the provided services. There is no co-pay for Medicare and Mr. Adams does not make any payment at this time. His diagnosis is benign hypertension. He will return on Thursday at 10:00 a.m. for a reexamination. Complete an insurance claim for a Level 3 Office Visit (with a -25 modifier for the additional EKG procedure), and an EKG with interpretation.

JOB 1-4

Jordan Connell calls to schedule his annual physical (99396). An appointment is made with Dr. Heath for Wednesday, March 6, at 2:30 p.m. Schedule the appointment, allowing 45 minutes for an established patient.

Because there are no patients scheduled until 1 p.m., it is a good time to process the mail and to complete any other paperwork.

JOB 1-5

A letter came from the bank indicating that the $71 check received on 3/1 from Jonathan Gibson did not clear the bank due to insufficient funds. The procedure in this instance is to pull the ledger card, place it over the day sheet, and reenter the charge on the ledger card (which automatically copies onto the day sheet; refer back to Figure 1-21). Also, place a call to Mr. Gibson to inform him of the nonsufficient funds (NSF) notice. If you are unable to reach Mr. Gibson, leave a message asking him to contact the office. Do not leave a message about the returned check as this is private information. There was no miscellaneous charge from the bank. Mr. Gibson's ledger card is returned to the accounts receivable section, awaiting payment after processing this procedure.

JOB 1-6

Dolores Perez, an established patient, walks into the office to make a $50.00 payment in cash on her account. Pull the ledger card and attach the shingle of receipts, enter the payment, and calculate the balance owed. Give Mrs. Perez a receipt and return the ledger card to the file. Be sure to enter the cash payment in the deposit record section of the day sheet.

JOB 1-7

Dr. Heath has given you the charges for Nancy Talbot, an established patient, who was hospitalized at Community General Hospital, 4000 Brand Blvd, Douglasville, NY 01234. Pull her ledger card to process the charges (refer back to Figure 1-23). Neither a superbill nor a receipt needs to be filled out because the claim will be sent to the insurance carrier. Check on the back of the ledger card to be sure that Mrs. Talbot's signature is on file. Mrs. Talbot was admitted to the hospital on February 10, with a diagnosis of gastroenteritis (558.9) and was discharged on February 13. Complete an insurance claim for Mrs. Talbot's hospitalization charges as shown in the example in **Figure 2-1**, but hold off submitting the claim until after her appointment in the office tomorrow. The two claims can then be sent together on one form.

1500

HEALTH INSURANCE CLAIM FORM

APPROVED BY NATIONAL UNIFORM CLAIM COMMITTEE 08/05

PICA ☐☐☐ | | PICA ☐☐☐

1. MEDICARE [X] (Medicare #) **MEDICAID** ☐ (Medicaid #) **TRICARE CHAMPUS** ☐ (Sponsor's SSN) **CHAMPVA** ☐ (Member ID#) **GROUP HEALTH PLAN** ☐ (SSN or ID) **FECA BLK LUNG** ☐ (SSN) **OTHER** ☐ (ID)

1a. INSURED'S I.D. NUMBER (For Program in Item 1)
123998099B

2. PATIENT'S NAME (Last Name, First Name, Middle Initial)
ANDERSON, KAY, T

3. PATIENT'S BIRTH DATE MM 07 DD 31 YY 1944 **SEX** M ☐ F [X]

4. INSURED'S NAME (Last Name, First Name, Middle Initial)

5. PATIENT'S ADDRESS (No., Street)
100 STATE STREET

6. PATIENT RELATIONSHIP TO INSURED
Self [X] Spouse ☐ Child ☐ Other ☐

7. INSURED'S ADDRESS (No., Street)

CITY DOUGLASVILLE **STATE** NY

8. PATIENT STATUS
Single [X] Married ☐ Other ☐
Employed ☐ Full-Time Student ☐ Part-Time Student ☐

CITY | **STATE**

ZIP CODE 01234 **TELEPHONE** (Include Area Code) (123)555-7091

ZIP CODE | **TELEPHONE** (Include Area Code) ( )

9. OTHER INSURED'S NAME (Last Name, First Name, Middle Initial)
ANDERSON, KAY, T

10. IS PATIENT'S CONDITION RELATED TO:

11. INSURED'S POLICY GROUP OR FECA NUMBER

a. OTHER INSURED'S POLICY OR GROUP NUMBER
12398099

a. EMPLOYMENT? (Current or Previous) YES ☐ NO ☐

a. INSURED'S DATE OF BIRTH MM DD YY **SEX** M ☐ F ☐

b. OTHER INSURED'S DATE OF BIRTH MM 07 DD 31 YY 1944 **SEX** M ☐ F [X]

b. AUTO ACCIDENT? YES ☐ NO ☐ **PLACE** (State)

b. EMPLOYER'S NAME OR SCHOOL NAME

c. EMPLOYER'S NAME OR SCHOOL NAME

c. OTHER ACCIDENT? YES ☐ NO ☐

c. INSURANCE PLAN NAME OR PROGRAM NAME

d. INSURANCE PLAN NAME OR PROGRAM NAME
MEDICAID

10d. RESERVED FOR LOCAL USE

d. IS THERE ANOTHER HEALTH BENEFIT PLAN?
[X] YES ☐ NO *If yes,* return to and complete item 9 a-d.

READ BACK OF FORM BEFORE COMPLETING & SIGNING THIS FORM.
12. PATIENT'S OR AUTHORIZED PERSON'S SIGNATURE I authorize the release of any medical or other information necessary to process this claim. I also request payment of government benefits either to myself or to the party who accepts assignment below.

SIGNED SIGNATURE ON FILE   DATE

13. INSURED'S OR AUTHORIZED PERSON'S SIGNATURE I authorize payment of medical benefits to the undersigned physician or supplier for services described below.

SIGNED SIGNATURE ON FILE

14. DATE OF CURRENT: MM DD YY ILLNESS (First symptom) OR INJURY (Accident) OR PREGNANCY(LMP)

15. IF PATIENT HAS HAD SAME OR SIMILAR ILLNESS. GIVE FIRST DATE MM DD YY

16. DATES PATIENT UNABLE TO WORK IN CURRENT OCCUPATION FROM MM DD YY TO MM DD YY

17. NAME OF REFERRING PROVIDER OR OTHER SOURCE
17a.
17b. NPI

18. HOSPITALIZATION DATES RELATED TO CURRENT SERVICES FROM MM 02 DD 15 YY TO MM 02 DD 18 YY

19. RESERVED FOR LOCAL USE

20. OUTSIDE LAB? YES ☐ NO ☐ **$ CHARGES**

21. DIAGNOSIS OR NATURE OF ILLNESS OR INJURY (Relate Items 1, 2, 3 or 4 to Item 24E by Line)
1. 496
2. ___
3. ___
4. ___

22. MEDICAID RESUBMISSION CODE ORIGINAL REF. NO.

23. PRIOR AUTHORIZATION NUMBER

24. A. DATE(S) OF SERVICE From MM DD YY	To MM DD YY	B. PLACE OF SERVICE	C. EMG	D. PROCEDURES, SERVICES, OR SUPPLIES (Explain Unusual Circumstances) CPT/HCPCS	MODIFIER	E. DIAGNOSIS POINTER	F. $ CHARGES	G. DAYS OR UNITS	H. EPSDT Family Plan	I. ID. QUAL.	J. RENDERING PROVIDER ID. #
1	02 15		21		99221		1	145 00	1		NPI	
2	02 16	02 17	21		99231		1	79 00	2		NPI	
3	02 18		21		99238		1	145 00	1		NPI	
4											NPI	
5											NPI	
6											NPI	

25. FEDERAL TAX I.D. NUMBER SSN ☐ EIN [X]
00-1234560

26. PATIENT'S ACCOUNT NO.

27. ACCEPT ASSIGNMENT? (For govt. claims, see back) [X] YES ☐ NO

28. TOTAL CHARGE $ 448 00

29. AMOUNT PAID $

30. BALANCE DUE $ 448 00

31. SIGNATURE OF PHYSICIAN OR SUPPLIER INCLUDING DEGREES OR CREDENTIALS (I certify that the statements on the reverse apply to this bill and are made a part thereof.)
SIGNATURE ON FILE

SIGNED   DATE

32. SERVICE FACILITY LOCATION INFORMATION
COMMUNITY GENERAL HOSPITAL
4000 BRAND BLVD
DOUGLASVILLE, NY 01234
a. 9997794511 b.

33. BILLING PROVIDER INFO & PH # (123)456-7890
DOUGLASVILLE MEDICINE ASSOCIA
5076 BRAND BLVD, STE 401
DOUGLASVILLE, NY 01234
a. 9995010111 b.

NUCC Instruction Manual available at: www.nucc.org   APPROVED OMB-0938-0999 FORM CMS-1500 (08/05)

FIGURE 2-1: Completed Insurance Claim for Hospital Charges. (Centers for Medicare and Medicaid Services.)

JOB 1-8

The letter carrier brings the mail, which contains a letter with $1.15 postage due. You pay this out of petty cash and record the amount on the day sheet. (Most offices have cash vouchers that would be filled out at this time. They are not included in this simulation.)

JOB 1-9

A check came in the mail from Medicare for $352.09. Process the payments for Walter Adams, Jessie Montgomery, and Dorothy Perez, referring to the explanation of benefits (EOB) provided in **Figure 2-2**.

JOB 1-10

Set up the check register sheet following the directions listed in **Procedure 9** in the Reference Manual. Using the check register sheet, place the shingles of checks over the appropriate line and issue check No. 479 to Straub & Son Remodeling Company in payment for the invoice shown in **Figure 2-3**. Record the amount in the column for Maintenance and Repairs in the check register. The Beginning Bank Balance is $1,952.80. Enter the check number, the date paid, and the amount paid on the invoice.

				MEDICARE				
PT NAME	**DOS**	**PROC**	**BILLED**	**ALLOWED**	**DEDUCTIBLE**	**CO-INS**	**WRITEOFF**	**PROV PD**
Adams, Walter	1/22	99221	145.00	92.33	0.00	18.47	52.67	73.86
	1/23-1/25	99231	237.00	117.21	0.00	23.44	119.79	93.77
	1/26	99238	145.00	92.33	0.00	18.47	52.67	73.86
TOTALS			**527.00**	**301.87**	**0.00**	**60.38**	**225.13**	**241.49**
Montgomery, Jesse	2/6	99213	111.00	69.13	0.00	13.83	41.87	55.30
TOTALS			**111.00**	**69.13**	**0.00**	**13.83**	**41.87**	**55.30**
Perez, Dorothy	1/31	99212	80.00	61.00	0.00	13.80	19.00	47.20
TOTALS			**80.00**	**61.00**	**0.00**	**13.80**	**19.00**	**47.20**
Claim information forwarded to: BCBS								
						TOTAL PAID TO PROVIDER		**352.09**

© Cengage Learning 2013

FIGURE 2-2: Medicare EOB.

STRAUB AND SON REMODELING COMPANY

67 Cottonwood Drive • Douglasville, NY 01234 • 123/555-1111

To: L.D. Heath, M.D.   Invoice # 167
      Douglasville Medicine Associates   Date: February 28, —
      5076 Brand Blvd, Suite 401
      Douglasville, NY 01234

- -

Install medical cabinet	5 hrs labor @ 15.50/hr		$77.50
1 Dark oak cabinet		*pd* ck #479 3/4/— $550.14	445.89
	Tax on supplies		26.75
	TOTAL		$ 550.14

© Cengage Learning 2013

FIGURE 2-3: Invoice from Straub and Son Remodeling Company.

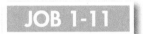

JOB 1-11

Issue check No. 480 to Diamond State Medical for supplies, using the invoice in **Figure 2-4**.

Diamond State Medical

2125 Creekside Drive
Newark, DE 19711
(302) 444-9908

Account No.: 270-54   Invoice No.: 3412

L.D. Heath, M.D.
Douglasville Medicine Associates
5076 Brand Blvd, Suite 401
Douglasville, NY 01234

Statement Date: 2/27/—

QTY.	UNIT	CAT. NUMBER	DESCRIPTION	UNIT PRICE	AMOUNT
1	100/BX	SC601175	SYR INSULIN 1ML	13.95	13.95
8	100/BX	SH501400	SYR TB 1ML	12.25	98.00
8	100/BX	SH250354	NEEDLE 26G × $^3/_8$"	7.95	63.60
2	100/BX	SH750510	NEEDLE 25G × $^5/_8$"	7.95	15.90
			Subtotal		$191.45
			State Tax (6%)		11.49
			Total—Pay this Amount		$202.94

© Cengage Learning 2013

FIGURE 2-4: Invoice from Diamond State Medical.

The office is closed from 12:00 to 1:00 p.m. The answering service will answer any calls and take messages.

JOB 1-12

After lunch, you call the answering service for messages and find out that Eric Garcia has cancelled his 1:45 p.m. appointment for today. You call him back and reschedule for Thursday at 9:00 a.m. Dr. Heath has asked you to schedule a blood sugar test for Mr. Garcia for this visit. Because Mr. Garcia has diabetes mellitus, type 2, and must fast for this test, an early morning appointment would be best for him. In the appointment book, you would erase Eric Garcia's name to allow that time slot to be filled, even at this late date, and reenter it for Thursday, March 7, at 9:00 a.m. Depending on the office policy, documentation of the cancelled appointment may be entered in the patient's medical record. Many times the cancelled appointment is recorded in the patient's medical record only if the appointment is not rescheduled.

JOB 1-13

Maureen Michaels, a new patient, arrives for her 1:00 p.m. appointment about 15 minutes late. You check with Dr. Heath, who says he will still see the patient. The scheduling in the office will not fall behind because Eric Garcia had cancelled his appointment, allowing flexibility in the schedule and giving Dr. Heath time to see Ms. Michaels even though she arrived late for her appointment. Ms. Michaels has just moved to New York and has

Ms. Maureen B. Michaels
43 Mountain Church Road
Douglasville, NY 01234
(123) 555-3288

Date of birth: 6/26/1971

Soc. Sec. No.: 545-22-3908

Nearest relative: David Michaels (spouse)

Employer: Not employed

Spouse's employer: Michaels Industries
Same address
(123) 555-2745

Insurance: Self-pay

Release: Signature on file

HIPAA form: Signed and acknowledged; copy given to patient

a history of asthmatic bronchitis. She wants to begin seeing Dr. Heath regularly. She would like to discuss budget payments because she has no insurance. The office policy is to accept budget payments if the payments are made on a regular basis. Ms. Michaels is pleased with these arrangements. She writes a check for today's charge of $147.00 for a Level 2 Office Visit. Issue her a receipt. There is no insurance form to complete.

JOB 1-14

Raymond O'Neill comes in for his regular twice-weekly checkup scheduled for 2:00 p.m. He has tested positive for HIV (the virus that causes AIDS) and comes in every Monday and Thursday at 2 p.m. for clinical and treatment evaluation. Today he is complaining of a cough and is diagnosed as having acute bronchitis. Charge his account for a Level 2 Office Visit and a chest x-ray in the office. He will be sent to the laboratory for a CBC with differential. Medicaid will be billed for these charges. Dr. Heath must accept the allowable amounts because he is a participating provider in this government insurance plan. Because of the sensitive nature of Mr. O'Neill's condition, his diagnosis (HIV-positive) will not be written in the appointment book or on the patient list. The office has set up a code or a method of identifying sensitive conditions such as HIV-positive status or AIDS by stating "return visit" with no diagnosis entered or by entering a code number. The method used is up to the discretion of the individual facility and the physician. Complete an insurance claim using acute bronchitis (466.0) as the diagnosis. The procedure codes include a Level 2 Office Visit, and a chest x-ray.

JOB 1-15

Michelle McLoud, an established patient, comes to the office for her 2:15 p.m. visit complaining about pain in her right ear. Mrs. McLoud is diagnosed with otitis media. She is charged a Level 2 Office Visit and pays the $80 charge with cash. Prepare a receipt, and schedule a return appointment for Monday, March 11, at 4:00 p.m.

JOB 1-16

Christopher Likens, an established patient, calls to make an appointment for tomorrow. He first saw Dr. Heath last Thursday, after experiencing chest pain and dyspnea. You tell him his x-ray has been evaluated, and you make an appointment for 11:00 a.m. on Tuesday, March 5. Mr. Likens' telephone number is (123) 555-3698.

Dr. Heath leaves the office at 3:00 p.m. for the day to make hospital visits. Before he leaves the office, remind Dr. Heath of the dinner meeting tonight at 5:00 p.m. and the staff breakfast tomorrow from 9:00 to 10:00 a.m.

JOB 1-17

Total the day sheet and prove your totals. Previous page amounts are as follows:

Col. A   = $515.20

Col. B-1 = $483.00

Col. B-2 = $60.03

Col. C   = $4,266.96

Col. D   = $4,294.79

In the Accounts Receivable Control, the Previous Day's Total is $3,676.40. In the Accounts Receivable Proof, the Accts. Rec. 1st of Month is $3,704.23. The Beginning Cash On Hand in the Cash Control box was $45.00 and the $1.15 labeled "postage due" will be subtracted from the $45.00. (Refer back to Figure 1-23, totaling the day sheet.)

JOB 1-18

Complete the deposit slip, record the deposit in the check register, and calculate the current bank balance. (Refer back to Figures 1-24 and 1-25, check endorsement and preparing the deposit slip.)

JOB 1-19

Because there appears to be a break in the schedule, use this time to prepare the patient list for tomorrow. Use the form provided in the forms section in the back of this book.

JOB 1-20

Complete the appropriate Daily Checkup form provided in the forms section in the back of the book.

MARCH				
4	5	6	7	8
Monday	**Tuesday**	Wednesday	Thursday	Friday

Your second day begins. As you check Dr. Heath's calendar, you note that he will be at a hospital staff breakfast until 10:00 a.m. and leaving for a lecture at the Douglasville Community College at 4:00 p.m. Place the medical records and a copy of the patient list on his desk. Then call the answering service and follow through as needed on any messages. Open the mail and sort, as previously directed. Post the incoming checks and complete any unfinished insurance forms until it is time for the first patient to arrive.

JOB 2-1

In today's mail, an Aetna insurance payment for Mary McDonald's January 8–12 hospitalization was received. Using the provided EOB in **Figure 2-5**, post the payment of $502.00 on the ledger card and the day sheet. Mrs. McDonald's responsibility is $25.00 and the bill will be sent to her.

JOB 2-2

Dr. Heath receives another check in the mail for $91.00 from FlexiHealth PPO for Leonard Mathers's 2/14 office visit **(see Figure 2-6)**. Record this transaction on the day sheet and ledger card. Mr. Mathers will be sent a statement showing the balance on his account.

AETNA						
Member's Name	DOS	Units	Procedure Code	Billed	Member Responsibility	Paid to Physician
Mary McDonald	1/8	1	99221	145.00	25.00	120.00
	1/9-1/11	3	99231	237.00	0.00	237.00
	1/12	1	99238	145.00	0.00	145.00
TOTALS				527.00	25.00	502.00

FIGURE 2-5: Aetna EOB for Mary McDonald.

FLEXIHEALTH PPO						
Member's Name	DOS	Units	Procedure Code	Billed	Member Responsibility	Paid to Physician
Leonard Mathers	2/14	1	99213	111.00	20.00	91.00
TOTALS				111.00	20.00	91.00

FIGURE 2-6: FlexiHealth PPO EOB for Leonard Mathers.

MEDICAID							
Member's Name	DOS	Units	Procedure Code	Billed	Non-Allowed Charges	Member Responsibility	Paid to Physician
Raymond O'Neill	2/28	1	99212	80.00	32.00	0.00	48.00
	2/28	1	71020	54.00	11.37	0.00	42.63
TOTALS				**134.00**	**43.37**	**0.00**	**90.63**

© Cengage Learning 2013

FIGURE 2-7: Medicaid EOB for Raymond O'Neill.

JOB 2-3

A Medicaid check for Raymond O'Neill was received in the amount of $90.63 for Mr. O'Neill's 2/28 Level 2 Office Visit and chest x-ray (see Figure 2-7).

The amount submitted to Medicaid was a total of $134.00. The office visit charge was $80.00 and Medicaid allowed $48.00. The $32.00 represents the difference between the amount submitted ($80.00) and the amount allowed ($48.00). The charge for the x-ray was $54.00 and the allowed amount was $43.37. The $11.37 represents the nonallowable charge for the x-ray. The total payment of $90.63 is entered in the payment column; the nonallowed charges of $43.37 are entered in the adjustment column and will be written off, and a total of $134.00 ($90.63 + $43.37) is subtracted from the previous balance of $268.00, now giving the patient a new balance of $134.00. Post the payments on the ledger card and day sheet.

> $80.00 + 54.00 = $134.00 total submitted to Medicaid (Col. A)
> −48.00 + 42.63 = 90.63 total Medicaid allowed amount (amount paid) (Col. B1)
> 43.37 adjusted amount for office visit (write-off amount) (Col. B2)
> Balance Col. C = 0

JOB 2-4

Dr. Heath receives a bill for staff dues at the hospital (see Figure 2-8). Write check No. 481 to Mercer General Hospital for payment of Dr. Heath's staff dues and record it in the check register.

JOB 2-5

Dr. Heath also receives a bill from City Answering Service (see Figure 2-9). Write check No. 482 for payment in full and record it in the check register.

MERCER GENERAL HOSPITAL

L. D. Heath, M.D.   March 1, —
5076 Brand Blvd, Suite 401
Douglasville, NY 01234

STAFF DUES. $200.00

Includes dues, library fees, and staff social functions.
Please make your check payable to: Mercer General Hospital and
MAIL YOUR REMITTANCE BY MARCH 15 TO:

Mercer General Hospital
Attn: Paul Huang, M.D.
900 Hamilton Avenue
Douglasville, NY 01234

© Cengage Learning 2013

FIGURE 2-8: Invoice for Staff Dues.

CITY
ANSWERING   400 Pearl Street
SERVICE   Douglasville, NY 01234
                       (123) 555-3629

                                        February 27, —

                       SERVICE CHARGE   68.00
                       MESSAGE UNITS   11.60
                       OUTGOING CALLS   25.80
                       POSTAGE   .00
                       OTHER   .00
                       PREVIOUS BALANCE   .00
                                                 _____
                       TOTAL   105.40

Invoice 4734
To: L. D. Heath, M.D.
      5076 Brand Blvd, Suite 401
      Douglasville, NY 01234

A CHARGE OF 1½% PER MONTH • 18% PER ANNUM WILL BE MADE ON PAST DUE BALANCE.

© Cengage Learning 2013

FIGURE 2-9: Invoice from City Answering Service.

JOB 2-6

Mrs. Setsu Arimura comes in to make a payment. She gives you $111.00 cash toward her deductible for her visit on February 27 for abdominal pain, which Dr. Heath diagnosed as gastroenteritis. Mrs. Arimura has requested a superbill with information regarding the office visit and treatment.

Although both Mr. and Mrs. Arimura have health insurance, Mrs. Arimura has the primary insurance and the claim was sent to her insurance company first. Record this payment and prepare a superbill for Setsu Arimura. Record the payment on the day sheet, but not in the Business Analysis Summary Column, because the service was not provided today.

JOB 2-7

Susan Deng, an established patient, arrives for her 10:00 a.m. appointment complaining of a sore throat. Dr. Heath performs a rapid strep test. Complete a superbill for Mrs. Deng. She is self-pay so there is no insurance claim to prepare. Diagnosis: Acute pharyngitis; procedures: Level 3 Office Visit, rapid strep test (87880). Mrs. Deng paid $157 with a personal check.

JOB 2-8

A new patient, Anna Miller, arrives for her 10:15 a.m. appointment. Her chief complaint is a nonproductive cough. You give Mrs. Miller a patient information sheet to complete. Use the information provided to complete her ledger card.

Dr. Heath sees the patient for 45 minutes and has a chest x-ray done in the office. The physician diagnoses Mrs. Miller with acute bronchitis. Record the charges for the office visit (Level 2) and chest x-ray. Mrs. Miller needs to return to the office for a reexamination. Make an appointment for her for Friday, March 8, at 10:45 a.m.

Anna F. Miller
232 Bayberry Rd
Douglasville, NY 01234
(123) 555-4790

DOB: 9/18/1940

Soc. Sec. No.: 184-21-8864

Nearest relative: Michael Miller (spouse)

Employer: Retired

Insurance: Medicare

ID No.: 184-21-8864A
No secondary insurance

Release: Signature on file, accepts assignment

HIPAA form: Signed and acknowledged; copy given to patient

Start the insurance claim but hold off submitting the claim until after Friday's return visit; then the two claims can be sent together on one form. Remember to add the modifier -25 to the Office Visits for both days because other separate procedures such as a chest x-ray and venipuncture were done at the time of the office visit. Mrs. Miller has signed the necessary insurance consent forms to release information and to assign payment to the physician. These forms are now on file.

JOB 2-9

Bryan Lake calls. He is scheduled for a blood pressure check today at 11:15 a.m. Because of an emergency involving his father, Mr. Lake is unable to keep his appointment. Cancel this appointment as the patient requests. He decides to schedule his physical exam on March 8 at 11:00 a.m. Be sure to reschedule this appointment for 60 minutes now that it will be for a physical exam.

JOB 2-10

Dr. Heath sees Christopher Likens, an established patient, at 11:00 a.m. He is being reexamined for chest pain. Dr. Heath explains to Mr. Likens that his x-ray reveals pneumonia. The physician prescribes medication and rest. Schedule Mr. Likens for another appointment for Friday, March 8, at 9:45 a.m. Mr. Likens is on medical assistance (Medicaid). Submit an insurance claim for Mr. Likens. Diagnosis: pneumonia; procedure: Level 2 Office Visit. Give Mr. Likens a receipt, which lists the charges for today.

JOB 2-11

Nancy Talbot, an established patient, arrives for her 11:30 a.m. appointment. Dr. Heath saw Ms. Talbot last during February 10–13, when she was hospitalized for gastroenteritis. Today, the patient complains of severe diarrhea, which would be coded as an additional diagnosis. Dr. Heath advises the patient that she should be readmitted to the hospital for further testing, if the pain and diarrhea persist and the medication does not help. Ms. Talbot states that she will continue on the treatment plan and make her decision by her next visit. **Figure 2-10** shows a sample of the consent form for treatment that patients sign. The consent form is then kept in the patient's medical record. Charge Ms. Talbot for a Level 2 Office Visit. Because the insurance claim for Mrs. Talbot's hospitalization (2/10 to 2/13), which was posted yesterday, was not yet completed, add this visit to the insurance form. Give Mrs. Talbot a receipt for today's $20.00 cash co-payment. Before Mrs. Talbot leaves the office, remind her that she has a return visit on Monday, March 11, at 11:45 a.m. Give her a receipt with her appointment date marked.

Consent for Treatment

Date _____ Time _____

I authorize the performance of the following procedure(s)

_____ on

_____ to be performed by
                    (name of patient)

_____, MD.
                  (name of physician)

The following have been explained to _____ by Dr. _____.
                                                              (name of physician)

Nature of the procedure _____
                                              (describe procedure)

_____

For the purpose of _____

_____

The possible alternative methods of treatment are _____

_____

The possible consequences of the procedure are _____

_____

The risks involve the possibility of _____

_____

The possible complications of this procedure are _____

_____

    I have been advised of the serious nature of this procedure and have been further advised that if I desire a more detailed explanation of any of the foregoing or further information about the possible risks or complications, it will be given to me.
    I do not request a more detailed listing and explanation of the above information.

Signed: _____
                    (Patient/Parent/Guardian)

Witnessed by: _____

© Cengage Learning 2013

FIGURE 2-10: Consent for Treatment Form.

The office is closed from 12:00 to 1:00 p.m. The answering service will answer any calls and take messages.

JOB 2-12

Tracey Mascello, an established patient, arrives for her 1:00 p.m. visit for an influenza vaccine injection. Post the charges for the flu vaccine. ICD code: V04.81;

CPT codes: influenza virus vaccine (90658) and vaccine administration (90471). Mrs. Mascello is self-pay; prepare a receipt for her $61.00 personal check.

JOB 2-13

Dr. Heath sees Elena Blanco, a new patient, at 1:15 p.m. Dr. Heath performs a routine gynecological examination (V72.31), obtaining cells from the cervix for a Pap smear (88105). Mrs. Blanco thinks she may be pregnant because her last menstrual period (LMP) was January 5, 2013. Dr. Heath performs a pregnancy test. Mrs. Blanco pays the co-pay of $20 cash and requests a receipt. Record the necessary information for this visit. Note that although the Pap smear will be analyzed by an outside laboratory, a specimen handling charge (99000) is applied. Include on the posting transaction the pregnancy test and New Patient Preventative Visit (99385) as well. Complete an insurance claim for Mrs. Blanco.

Mrs. Elena R. Blanco
550 Federal City Road
Douglasville, NY 01234
(123) 555-2659

Date of birth: 4/30/1985

Soc. Sec. No.: 162-84-5559

Nearest relative: Paul Blanco (spouse)
Same address

Employer: Part-time employment at:
Douglasville Community College
Douglasville, NY 01234
(123) 555-7511

Insurance: Under Paul (husband)

Paul: DOB: 05/07/1984

Paul: Soc. Sec. No.: 042-15-7762

ID No.: 003475-1-98

Group No.: 00047532
FlexiHealth PPO (under Paul [husband])

Co-pay: $20

Release: Signature on file; accepts assignment

HIPAA form: Signed and ackmowledged; copy given to patient

JOB 2-14

At about 1:30 p.m., Joanna Phillips, an established patient, calls. Last week, while on vacation, she twisted her neck on an amusement park ride. She was treated by an emergency physician in Orlando, Florida. Her neck is really bothering her and she requests an appointment to have her neck pain reexamined. You give her a 3:00 p.m. appointment today.

JOB 2-15

At 2:15 p.m., Thomas P. Smith, an established patient, arrives for his visit to have his blood pressure rechecked and to receive his allergy injection. Post the charges for Mr. Smith and complete his insurance claim using the following information: Procedures: Level 2 Office Visit, allergy injection (95115); diagnosis: benign hypertension and allergic rhinitis. Mr. Smith pays the $10 co-pay in cash. Give him a receipt and schedule Mr. Smith for Monday, March 11, at 2:15 p.m. for a physical examination (allow 60 minutes).

JOB 2-16

Aimee Bradley is scheduled for 2:30 p.m. By 2:45 p.m. she still has not arrived for her appointment. She never called to change or cancel the appointment. A call placed to her cell phone and her home results in getting an answering machine. Document a "no-show" in the appointment book by circling the patient's name in red ink and enter the date of service and time of the appointment that was missed in the patient's medical record in red ink. Many offices will call the patient to check on them and perhaps reschedule the missed appointment.

JOB 2-17

Joanna Phillips arrives for her 3:00 p.m. office visit and is examined by Dr. Heath. Charge Ms. Phillips for a Level 2 Office Visit. She pays the $80 fee with a check and requests a receipt.

Dr. Heath leaves for his 4:00 p.m. lecture at Douglasville Community College. Because you are working to 5:00 p.m. and no more patients are scheduled for the day, it is a good time to finishing completing any insurance claims or finish posting any checks that came in the mail.

JOB 2-18

A $101.00 insurance claim check was received in the mail from Signal HMO for Alan Silverstein's 2/26 office visit. The balance on Mr. Silverstein's account was $91.00 because he paid $20.00 for the co-pay instead of the required $10.00, giving him a $10 credit on his account. The office manager asks you to post a refund of $10.00 on the ledger card and day sheet for Mr. Silverstein and she will prepare the check for Dr. Heath to sign.

JOB 2-19

Jonathan Gibson walks into the office to pay in cash the $71.00 remainder of his balance owed due to the NSF check that did not clear the bank. Post the payment and give Mr. Gibson a receipt.

JOB 2-20

Thomas Smith calls and asks if the physician can see his daughter, Heather, tomorrow because she is complaining of a sore throat. You give her a 9:00 a.m. appointment tomorrow, Wednesday, March 6.

JOB 2-21

Total the day sheet and prove your totals. Complete the deposit slip, record the deposit in the check register, and calculate the current bank balance.

JOB 2-22

Prepare the patient list for tomorrow.

JOB 2-23

Complete the appropriate Daily Checkup form.

MARCH				
4	5	**6**	7	8
Monday	Tuesday	**Wednesday**	Thursday	Friday

Dr. Heath is scheduled to begin seeing patients at 9:00 a.m. Place the pulled medical records on his desk with the patient list for the day.

JOB 3-1

Aimee Bradley calls and apologizes for missing her appointment yesterday and asks if she can be seen this morning. She says that her eyes are red and watery. You give her a 10:00 a.m. appointment.

JOB 3-2

Heather Smith arrives for her 9:00 a.m. appointment with her mother. She is the 11-year-old daughter of Thomas and Laurie Smith. In the pegboard system, all family members are included on one ledger card. Each member's name is entered into the reference section of the card to distinguish which member of the family is receiving treatment from the physician. Dr. Heath examines Heather and diagnoses her problem as purulent tonsillitis. Although tonsillitis is most often caused by a virus, it can be caused by bacteria such as *Streptococcus*, so Dr. Heath decides to perform a strep screen test to rule out a strep infection. Post the charges for Heather's visit: Established patient, child visit (99392), $50.00, and a strep screen (87081), $16.00. Give a receipt for the $10.00 cash co-pay. Complete an insurance claim for Heather. Although both Mr. and Mrs. Smith have health insurance, Mrs. Smith has the primary insurance (sent to her insurance company first) following the **Birthday Rule**. This rule states that when dealing with married parents of children and both parents have insurance, the parent whose birthday comes first in the year will provide the primary insurance for the child, and the other parent's insurance will be the secondary insurance (sent to this insurance company after the claim has been accepted or rejected by the primary insurance). Because Laurie Smith's birthday is in January and Thomas Smith's birthday is in September, Laurie's insurance becomes the primary insurance and Thomas Smith's insurance becomes the secondary insurance. Schedule a return appointment for Monday, March 11, at 10:45 a.m.

JOB 3-3

Leonard Mathers, an established patient, arrives for his appointment. He is complaining of indigestion and chest pain. Mr. Mathers pays today's co-pay and the co-pay owed from the previous visit (2/14) with a $40.00 personal check. Enter the charges: Level 3 Office Visit; EKG (93000); chest x-ray (71020) on the ledger card and the day sheet, giving Mr. Mathers a superbill, using gastroesophageal reflux (GERD) and chest pain as the diagnoses. The insurance claim will be completed by Dr. Heath's part-time office assistant. On the ledger, post the transaction of $20.00 to the amount owed from the last visit and give Mr. Mathers a receipt. On the next line, post today's charges and the $20.00 co-pay, completing the superbill.

JOB 3-4

Aimee Bradley, an established patient, arrives for her appointment, complaining of red, watery eyes. Dr. Heath diagnoses her symptoms as conjunctivitis. Aimee paid the $15 co-pay in cash and requests a superbill. Post the transaction for a Level 2 Office Visit. The insurance claim will be completed by Dr Heath's part-time office assistant.

JOB 3-5

Dr. Heath gives you the hospitalization dates for Isabel Durand, 1/26–1/31 at Community General Hospital. Post the charges as follows: diagnosis: COPD; procedure codes: hospital admission (1/26), 99221; four subsequent visits (1/27–1/30), 99231; hospital discharge (1/31), 99238. Complete the insurance claim. Mrs. Durand has both Medicare and Medicaid, government health insurance plans. Medicare is primary over Medicaid and therefore is the primary insurance. Once Medicare has paid its portion of the bill, the claim is sent on to Medicaid as the secondary or Medigap insurance. Medicaid may pay the Medicare deductibles and even the 20% portion of the medical charges not paid by Medicare, depending on the rules of the individual state.

JOB 3-6

Jessie Montgomery, an established patient, is scheduled for 10:30 a.m. for a recheck of her asthmatic bronchitis. Post the charges for today's visit Level 2 Office Visit on the ledger card and day sheet. Mrs. Montgomery requests a superbill to keep track of her visits.

JOB 3-7

Nancy Herbert, an established patient, arrives for her 11:15 a.m. appointment for a recheck of her urinary tract infection (UTI). Mrs. Herbert states that the burning on urination is getting worse. Dr. Heath performs a urine test with microscopy (81000) and also a test for blood sugar since Mrs. Herbert has diabetes mellitus, type 2. Charge Mrs. Herbert for a Level 3 Office Visit, blood sugar test, and urine test. Give Mrs. Herbert a superbill itemizing her services today. Complete her insurance claim and schedule an appointment for Monday, March 11, at 9:15 a.m.

Time is allowed in the morning in case of emergency appointments that might be needed. Today, 11:30 a.m.–12:00 p.m. is left open. Because no patients called to be seen during this time, you may use it to post any checks that were received in the mail.

JOB 3-8

The letter carrier brings the mail, which contains a letter with $1.25 postage due. You pay this out of petty cash and record the amount on the day sheet. (Most offices have cash vouchers that would be filled out at this time. They are not included in this simulation.)

JOB 3-9

You open and sort the mail. Included is a $20.00 check from Josephine Albertson for her 1/31 visit. Post the payment on the ledger card and day sheet. No receipt is necessary because her cancelled check will serve as her receipt.

JOB 3-10

Another check was received, for Eric Garcia's January 18 office visit. Record the $95.25 check from FlexiHealth PPO insurance company for Eric Garcia on his ledger card and the day sheet. Because Dr. Heath is a participating physician in FlexiHealth PPO, he agrees to the amount allowed by the insurance carrier, which is $95.25. The $14.75 is the adjustment portion of the bill and must be written off.

JOB 3-11

An EOB from FlexiHealth PPO came in today's mail with a check for Josephine Albertson's office visit on January 31 in the amount of $55.25. The adjustment is $4.75. Record this transaction on the ledger card and day sheet.

JOB 3-12

One of your responsibilities this week in Dr. Heath's office is to prepare the payroll for two employees. The first payroll check will be for Joseph M. Pinelli for maintenance work at Douglasville Medicine Associates. Mr. Pinelli worked 40 hours this week. His W-4 shows he is married and has two allowances. Joseph's rate of pay is $15.00 an hour. Record on the check the amount of his net pay and the amount of taxes withheld. Record these amounts on the check register under the four appropriate headings: Federal Withholding (Fed), State Withholding (State), Social Security (SS), and Medicare, and Net Payroll.

JOB 3-13

Prepare a payroll check for the part-time filing clerk, Sara C. Jackson. She worked 20 hours this week at $17.50 an hour. Her W-4 shows she is married and has two allowances. Record the amount of this check on the check register and the amount of withholdings in the appropriate columns.

The office is closed from 12:00 to 1:00 p.m. Remind Dr. Heath that he has a lunch seminar at the hospital today at 12:00 p.m. The answering service will answer any calls and take messages.

JOB 3-14

After lunch you check with the answering service to find that Pamela Cameron's lab work is completed. You call Ms. Cameron to remind her of her appointment for tomorrow at 10:15 a.m., March 7.

JOB 3-15

A payment of $60.00 was made by Francois Blanc because he thought his insurance company would not cover the bill. A check for $60.00 arrived in today's mail from Medicare Statewide insurance. Mr. Blanc now has a credit balance. The office manager asks you to post a refund on his ledger card and the day sheet. She will write the check and have Dr. Heath sign it.

JOB 3-16

At 2:30 p.m., Jordan Connell arrives for his wellness physical. Dr. Heath performs various tests for the complete physical (CP), which include an Hct, EKG, urinalysis without microscopy, and chest x-ray. Complete the ledger card and the day sheet. Mr. Connell pays his co-pay of $25 in cash; prepare a superbill.

JOB 3-17

Isabel Durand calls and would like to make an appointment for tomorrow, March 7, if there is an opening. She explains that she was released from the hospital for COPD and would like to see Dr. Heath. Schedule her for 10:45 a.m.

JOB 3-18

Total the day sheet and prove your totals.

JOB 3-19

Complete the deposit slip, record the deposit in the check register, and calculate the current bank balance.

JOB 3-20

Prepare the patient list for tomorrow.

JOB 3-21

Complete the appropriate Daily Checkup form.

MARCH				
4	5	6	7	8
Monday	Tuesday	Wednesday	**Thursday**	Friday

The daily slots left open for emergencies today are 1:30 p.m. and 1:45 p.m.

JOB 4-1

Today's first patient is Eric Garcia for reexamination (Level 2 Office Visit) of his diabetes mellitus. A blood sugar test was performed in the office. (Mr. Garcia was given an early morning appointment because this test required a fasting specimen.) Prepare a receipt for today's co-pay of $20.00 cash.

JOB 4-2

Margaret Chandler arrives to discuss the results of her test. Dr. Heath tells the patient that the tests confirmed the diagnosis of angina pectoris. Dr. Heath prescribes nitroglycerin tablets sublingually for pain and encourages her to rest and avoid overexertion. Mrs. Chandler will return in 2 weeks for a reexamination. The patient will call to schedule this appointment. She makes a $20 co-pay in cash and requests a receipt.

JOB 4-3

Walter Adams arrives for his 10:00 a.m. appointment. After he sees the physician, you explain his account balance to him; he gives you a check for $60 and requests a receipt. Dr. Heath has asked him to call next week if he is having any trouble. His diagnosis is benign hypertension. Post today's transactions for a Level 2 Office Visit.

JOB 4-4

Pamela Cameron comes in for the results of her lab work, which show an iron deficiency. Dr. Heath orders a CBC to be performed at an outside laboratory. She wants to know if the medication, which was started on Monday, has been effective. Charge Ms. Cameron for a Level 3 Office Visit and give her an appointment on Monday, March 11, at 3:15 p.m. There is no payment due at this time.

JOB 4-5

Isabel Durand arrives for her appointment. Several minutes later she begins having severe chest pains and trouble breathing. Another worker immediately takes Ms. Durand to an examination room in a wheelchair while you inform Dr. Heath. He tells you to call the hospital for an ambulance while he performs an EKG. It shows Ms. Durand is having atrial fibrillation and is taken to the hospital to be admitted.

Complete Ms. Durand's ledger card and the day sheet, charging her only for the EKG. (Most insurance plans will not pay for an office visit and a hospital visit on the same day.) Since the hospital admission will entail a more comprehensive work-up by the physician, this procedure will be the one charged to the patient rather than the brief office visit. The hospital admission charge will be put through the board (day sheet) at a later time. No receipt is needed at this time because the claim will be sent to the insurance carrier by the medical office assistant.

JOB 4-6

Xao Chang, an established patient, arrives for his CP at 11:00 a.m. Charge Mr. Chang for a wellness visit. Since Mr. Chang is over 65 years of age you will use the CPT code 99397 for the wellness CP. The ICD code is a V-code, V70.0. Post the transactions for a CP, EKG, and a urinalysis without microscopy. Mr. Chang will be sent to an outside laboratory for a complete CBC so there is no charge or paperwork to be completed for that procedure. Give Mr. Chang a receipt for his $15 co-pay in cash. Make an appointment for Monday, March 11 at, 4:30 p.m. to go over the results of his tests. Mr. Chang's insurance form will be completed by the medical office assistant.

The office is closed from 12:00 noon to 1:00 p.m. The answering service will answer any calls and take messages. After lunch, you call the answering service to see if there have been any messages. You are told that Dolores Perez will be 20 minutes late because of a change in the bus schedule. Give this information to Dr. Heath.

JOB 4-7

A check came in the mail from FlexiHealth PPO for payment of Josephine Albertson's 7/10 office visit. Post the transaction on the ledger card and the day sheet as follows: $55.25 payment; $4.75 adjustment. No receipt is necessary for the third-party payer.

JOB 4-8

Dr. Heath gives you the daily convalescent homes charges for Francois Blanc for the three visits (99307) on 3/5–3/7 Post the transactions on the ledger card and the day sheet. Complete the insurance claim for 3/5–3/7. His diagnosis is COPD and dehydration. Mr. Blanc resides at the Retirement Inn Nursing Home, 890 Millennium Way, Douglasville, NY 01234. In the Business Analysis Summary on the day sheet, record the charges in a new column labeled Outside Services.

JOB 4-9

Deanna Hartsfeld arrives for her appointment at 1:15 p.m. Today Mrs. Hartsfeld is complaining of frequent headaches. Dr. Heath checks her blood pressure and it is elevated. He decides to check her cholesterol level. Post the charges for a Level 3 Office Visit, and a test for cholesterol (82465). Give Mrs. Hartsfeld a receipt for her $15 cash co-pay.

JOB 4-10

Raymond O'Neill comes in for his biweekly checkup. No tests are scheduled for today. Remind him you will see him next Monday at the same time (2:00 p.m.). Post the transactions as a Level 2 Office Visit.

JOB 4-11

A check arrived from the bank listing an NSF $10.00 check for the account of Joanna Phillips. Post the transaction on the ledger card and day sheet to Mrs. Phillips' account. Be sure to call the patient and leave a message to call the office.

JOB 4-12

Ms. Perez arrives for her appointment. Dr. Heath tells her that her blood pressure level is slightly elevated and that she should remain on her diet of low-salt foods, continue taking the prescribed medication, and call for an appointment in 2 months. Dr. Heath orders a cholesterol test and says he will let her know the results. Although Dr. Heath accepts Medicare assignment, Ms. Perez has not yet met her yearly deductible. Charge Mrs. Perez for a Level 3 Office Visit and a cholesterol test. She gives you a check for $50.00, and you give her a receipt for her payment of $50.00. The medical office assistant will complete the insurance form for Mrs. Perez.

JOB 4-13

After Ms. Perez leaves, Dr. Heath goes to the hospital to check on Ms. Durand on the hospital unit. Record an initial hospital visit charge, 70 minutes (99223), on her ledger card and on the day sheet. No receipt or superbill is needed at this time. Remind Dr. Heath that he has a 5:00 p.m. staff meeting tonight.

JOB 4-14

Since Ms. Perez is the last patient of the day, total the day sheet and prove your totals.

JOB 4-15

Now complete the deposit slip.

JOB 4-16

Issue check No. 485 to Doctors' Medical Supply in payment of the invoice shown in **Figure 2-11**.

JOB 4-17

Issue check No. 486 to Central Cleaning Services in payment of the invoice shown in **Figure 2-12**. Then calculate the current bank balance by adding in today's deposit.

JOB 4-18

Now prepare the patient list for Friday.

DOCTORS' MEDICAL SUPPLY

3100 Vernon Boulevard
Douglasville, NY 01234
(123) 555-5501

Account # 007451   ORIGINAL INVOICE # 10358115

BILL TO	L. D. Heath, M.D. 5076 Brand Blvd, Suite 401 Douglasville, NY 01234

PURCHASE ORDER NUMBER	CREDIT CARD REFERENCE NO.		SALESPERSON	CONTACT	DATE
P.O. #6538			**MOLLY**	**SARA JACKSON**	**02/05/—**

QTY	UNIT	SHIPPED	BACK ORD'D	CAT. NUMBER	DESCRIPTION	UNIT PRICE	AMOUNT
6	BX	4		EM7853	LECTRO PADS/50/BX	8.75	35.00
12	BX	12		CC6350	EKG PAPER 2/RL/BX	6.30	75.60
5	BX	3		MM2420	MOUNT EKG 8 1/2 X 11 100/BX	28.95	86.85
4	EA	4		MB4121	SPECTRA EKG GEL 8 OZ.	2.50	10.00

CLAIMS FOR SHORTAGES MUST BE REPORTED
WITHIN 5 DAYS OF RECEIPT OF GOODS

PLEASE RETAIN THIS INVOICE. ANY ADDITIONAL
INVOICES ARE ONE DOLLAR EACH.

TERMS: NET 10 DAYS

SUBTOTAL	207.45
6% SALES TAX	12.45
3% HANDLING	6.22
TOTAL OF ORDER	226.12

PAYMENT DUE ON 03/15/—

NO RETURNS WITHOUT PRIOR AUTHORIZATION

FIGURE 2-11: Invoice from Doctors' Medical Supply.

CENTRAL CLEANING SERVICES
951 Kenmore Road
Douglasville, NY 01
(123) 555-2000

TO: L. D. Heath, M.D.
      5076 Brand Blvd, Suite 401
      Douglasville, NY 01234

Invoice Number: 4739
Invoice Date: March 1, —
Building Served: 420 Broad Street

Services Performed	Date	Amount
Monthly Cleaning: Floors, bathrooms, and windows	February, 19—	$120.00
TOTAL DUE		$120.00

FIGURE 2-12: Invoice from Central Cleaning Services.

JOB 4-19

Complete the appropriate Daily Checkup form.

MARCH				
4	5	6	7	**8**
Monday	Tuesday	Wednesday	Thursday	**Friday**

After pulling the medical records for the day and the patient list to put on Dr. Heath's desk, check the answering service for any messages.

JOB 5-1

Nancy Herbert left a message that she has a fever and a productive cough and would like to be seen today. You call her back and find out that her temperature is 102 degrees Fahrenheit, so you schedule her for 10:15 a.m. On today's appointment scheduling calendar, the time slots 10:15 a.m. and 10:30 a.m. were left open for patients who might call and request to be seen due to an illness that needed more immediate attention.

JOB 5-2

Dr. Heath examines Megan Caldwell for a UTI. Dysuria has decreased, and Dr. Heath suggests Ms. Caldwell continue to drink plenty of water. A urinalysis without microscopy is done. Charge a Level 2 Office Visit and a urinalysis without microscopy. Give Ms. Caldwell a receipt for her $20.00 cash co-pay.

JOB 5-3

Dr. Heath reexamines Christopher Likens for his pneumonia. Dr. Heath takes another chest x-ray to see if the pneumonia has resolved. Charge a Level 3 Office Visit and a chest x-ray. Give Mr. Likens a superbill listing today's services. Mr. Likens's insurance claim will be completed by the medical office assistant.

JOB 5-4

Nancy Herbert arrives for her 10:15 a.m. appointment. Dr. Heath collects a sputum specimen to send to the laboratory. There is a specimen handling charge for this procedure (99000). Dr. Heath also performs a rapid strep test. Mrs. Herbert still has a fever and Dr. Heath instructs Mrs. Herbert to rest and drink plenty of fluids. She is diagnosed with a fever of unknown origin. Post a Level 3 Office Visit, a rapid strep test, and a specimen handling charge. Mrs. Herbert pays $50.00 in cash toward her deductible. Give Mrs. Herbert a receipt. Mrs. Herbert already has an appointment on Monday, March 11, at 9:15 a.m. Add recheck on fever to the patient list for Monday. The medical office assistant will complete the insurance claim for today.

JOB 5-5

Andrew Jefferson appears at the office at 10:15 a.m. and states that he has a terrible sore throat. He has been seen by Dr. Schwartz in the past. Dr. Schwartz is not in today and Dr. Heath is covering so you tell Mr. Jefferson that Dr. Heath will see him at 10:30 a.m. Add him to your appointment book and patient list. Pull his medical record from the file and add it to the patient medical records for today. Note in the medical record that Dr. Heath is covering for Dr. Schwartz. Dr. Heath examines Mr. Jefferson and diagnoses his sore throat as viral infection. He performs a strep screen to rule out a strep throat. Charge Mr. Jefferson for a Level 3 Office Visit and a strep screen. Give him a receipt for his $20.00 cash co-pay. The medical office assistant will complete the insurance claim for today.

JOB 5-6

Patrick McDonald arrives at the office with a check to pay the balance of his wife's (Mary) account. He requests a receipt. Record the transaction. (Do not put the payment in the Business Analysis Summary column because the patient was not seen today.)

JOB 5-7

Anna Miller arrives for a reexamination of her recently diagnosed acute bronchitis. Ms. Miller states that she is still not feeling well and feels tired all the time. Dr. Heath examines her and orders that blood be drawn and sent to an outside lab for testing to check for anemia. Ms. Miller pays $50.00 toward her deductible by personal check and requests a receipt. The patient tells you that Dr. Heath has asked her to return on Monday, March 11. You give her an appointment for 9:45 a.m. Post the transactions for today, which includes a Level 3 Office Visit, a routine venipuncture (36415), and a specimen handling charge (99000). Complete today's insurance claim with Monday's claim. Remember to add the modifier -25 to the office visits for both days, since other separate procedures such as a chest x-ray and venipuncture were done at the time of the office visit.

JOB 5-8

Bryan Lake arrives for his 11:00 a.m. appointment. Dr. Heath performs a CP examination, including a urinalysis without microscopy, chest x-ray, and EKG. He orders a blood test for which blood must be drawn, a routine venipuncture, and sent to an outside lab (specimen handling charge). This annual examination is required by his employer. Mr. Lake presents a signed insurance form from his company, releasing medical information and allowing payment directly to Dr. Heath. The medical office assistant will complete the insurance claim. Give Mr. Lake a receipt for his $25.00 cash co-pay. Because the employer required the physical examination, Mr. Lake will be reimbursed by his employer when he submits the receipt for the co-pay.

The office is closed from 12:00 to 1:00 p.m. The answering service will answer any calls and take messages.

JOB 5-9

The first patient is not scheduled until 2:00 p.m.; you will have time to open the mail. Today Dr. Heath receives an invoice from Englewood Accounting Services **(see Figure 2-13)**. Write a check for this amount and record it in the Expense Distribution column headed Miscellaneous. On the line where you record the check, print "Tax Returns" again in the Description column, to the left of the payment amount. This will clearly identify this category of expense.

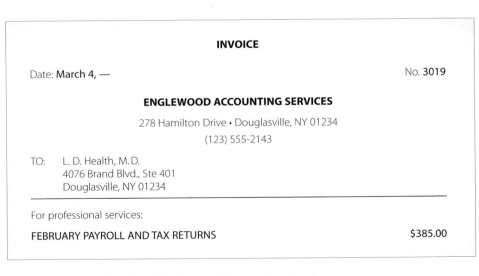

INVOICE

Date: **March 4, —**   No. **3019**

ENGLEWOOD ACCOUNTING SERVICES

278 Hamilton Drive • Douglasville, NY 01234

(123) 555-2143

TO: L. D. Health, M.D.
      4076 Brand Blvd., Ste 401
      Douglasville, NY 01234

For professional services:

FEBRUARY PAYROLL AND TAX RETURNS $385.00

FIGURE 2-13: Invoice from Englewood Accounting Services.

JOB 5-10

A second invoice arrives from the Tri-State Electric Company (**see Figure 2-14**). Write a check for this amount and record it as needed in the check register.

JOB 5-11

Walter Adams calls and cancels his 2:00 p.m. office visit. He has to cancel because his son cannot drive him to the appointment. He will reschedule when he can confirm transportation.

JOB 5-12

Post the personal check for $40.00 that arrives in the mail from Jessie Montgomery toward her account.

TRI-STATE ELECTRIC COMPANY
P.O. Box 7201
Tullytown, PA 19007

THIS IS YOUR BILL

Account Number 34-10-3489

....

DETACH HERE AND RETURN THIS PORTION WITH YOUR PAYMENT

BILLING INFORMATION

SERVICE TO:
L. D. Heath, M.D.
4076 Brand Blvd, Ste 401
Douglasville, NY 01234

Your account number is 34-10-3489.
If you have any questions about this bill, please contact us before the due date, by telephone at 215-555-5712 or by writing to P.O. Box 7201, Tullytown, PA, 19007.

Statement of account: Billing date February 28, —.

Previous balance (Recent payments not shown will appear on your next bill.)		218.97
Payment February 14 — Thank you		−218.97

Meter reading information and new charge rate RH

To Feb 22 Actual Reading	79005		
From Jan 17 Actual Reading	75811		
Kilowatt-Hours Billed (kWh)	3194	Base Rate	302.53

FIGURE 2-14: Invoice from Tri-State Electric Company.

JOB 5-13

You receive a $120.00 check from Medicaid for Christopher Likens's office visit and chest x-ray of February 28. The charge was $165.00 and Medicaid allowed $120.00. Dr. Heath must accept the Medicaid-allowed charges. Record the transaction.

JOB 5-14

A check for $99.25 came from Medicare Statewide for Nancy Herbert's March 6 visit. The adjustment is $32.75. Because Mrs. Herbert has a $10.00 co-pay with her Advantage Medicare plan, she will be responsible for the remaining $10.00 for that office visit. Post the payment and adjustment. She will be billed at a later time.

JOB 5-15

A check arrives from the After Hours Collection Agency for Helen Baldwin's overdue account of $296.00. Post the payment check for $177.60 on the ledger card and the day sheet. The collection agency (CA) takes a commission of 40% ($118.40) on the amount they collect and Dr. Heath's office receives 60% ($177.60). The $177.60 is entered in the payment column and the $118.40 is entered in the adjustment column, because that is the amount Dr. Heath will not be able to collect as it was the payment to the CA (refer back to Figure 1-21).

Dr. Heath leaves for the hospital at 4:00 p.m. for hospital rounds.

JOB 5-16

Total the day sheet and prove your totals.

JOB 5-17

Complete the deposit slip, record the deposit in the check register, and calculate the current bank balance.

JOB 5-18

Total all columns of the check register.

JOB 5-19

Complete the patient list for Monday.

JOB 5-20

Complete Friday's Daily Checkup.

JOB 5-21

Complete the Weekly Checkup.

You have survived! You have now completed all the work in the pegboard portion of this simulation. Even though you spent only one workweek in the physician's office, you have a better awareness and understanding of the responsibilities of being a medical office professional. Before leaving today and starting your weekend, check to make sure you have assembled all your work.

Enjoy your weekend—you deserve it!

SECTION 3

COMPUTER JOBS

Now that you have successfully completed 5 days in a medical office using the pegboard system, it is now time to transfer the medical record and bookkeeping knowledge learned in the pegboard system to the computer system. In this simulation, you will be using Medical Office Simulation Software (MOSS) 2.0, a simulated practice management software program. This program is on the CD-ROM within this package, and you will need to install the program on your computer to complete the following jobs. Use the directions in **Section 4, MOSS Installation and Setup Instructions** prior to starting the jobs.

The pegboard and computer system are very similar; both programs use the same information gathered from the patient at the time of registration and during patient visits. In order for either system to function properly, attention must be paid to details and accuracy.

Many offices employ computers to aid the medical office professional in completing front office procedures. Practice management software is available to assist office personnel in the following tasks:

- Creating and updating patient ledger cards
- Keeping track of appointments
- Producing a patient list
- A daily log of patient accounting transactions
- Posting payments to accounts receivable
- Preparing patient statements
- Preparing superbills and receipts
- Producing hard copies of insurance forms
- Transmitting electronic insurance claims
- Writing checks
- Keeping track of accounts payable

Electronic health record (EHR) software or word processing programs can be a great help in maintaining medical records and patient histories, recording physicians' progress notes, determining patient eligibility for insurance coverage, and carrying on correspondence. Computer programs are also available to produce labels for mailing, specimen identification, and many other tasks.

The computerized office has many advantages, especially:

- *Data management.* It is easy to enter and change data.

- *Search functionality.* It allows for simple storage and retrieval of information.

- *Printing and duplicate copies.* It offers the ability to print out multiple copies of data.

- *Data integrity.* Fewer errors are introduced than when using manual methods.

Potential difficulties with computerization include:

- *Breaches of security.* The confidentiality of medical records must be maintained. Only authorized personnel should be allowed access to data.

- *High costs.* Equipment such as computers, printers, and modems can be very costly, especially at the outset. Computer hardware and software may become obsolete in several years and should be replaced or upgraded on a regular basis. In addition, there are training costs associated with the computerized office.

- *Downtime.* Like any machines, computers can break down or malfunction. Proper maintenance is needed to minimize such problems.

The write-it-once system may be used instead of or in conjunction with computers in the medical office.

JOB 6-1 | SETTING UP THE MATRIX

One of the first tasks to be done is to set up the matrix of the appointment book. Setting up the matrix involves marking off the times when the physician is not available to see patients, when the office is not scheduling patients, or when the office is closed.

1. Open MOSS. Your username and password ("Student1") are already loaded for you. Click OK **(see Figure 3-1)**. You are now at the Main Menu screen.

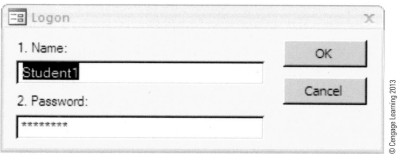

FIGURE 3-1: Logon Screen of MOSS.

2. From the Main Menu, click *Appointment Scheduling*. The Practice Schedule calendar will appear on the screen. Notice that the lunch hour, 12:00 noon to 1:00 p.m. (60 minutes) is already blocked for the 1-hour lunch period.

3. Click *Block Calendar* at the bottom of the screen.

4. You will receive a prompt, asking if you want to create a new calendar block. Click *Yes*.

5. When the block calendar window appears, complete Fields 1–9 with the following information:

    a. **Field 1.** Description: Hospital Rounds

    b. **Field 2.** Start Date: 03/04/2013 (when you tab to the next field, note that the numeric date changes to Monday, March 04, 2013)

    c. **Field 3.** End Date: 03/18/2013 (when you tab to the next field, note that the numeric date changes to Monday, March 18, 2013)

    d. **Field 4.** Time: 3:00 p.m.

    e. **Field 5.** Duration: 120 minutes (select from the drop-down list)

    f. **Field 6.** Frequency: Weekly (select from the drop-down list)

    g. **Field 7.** No. of Blocks: this is autopopulated by the program (based on the start and end dates, and frequency)

    h. **Field 8.** Pertains to: L. D. Heath, MD (select from the drop-down list)

    i. **Field 9.** Note: leave blank

6. Review your work with **Figure 3-2**. Click *Save*.

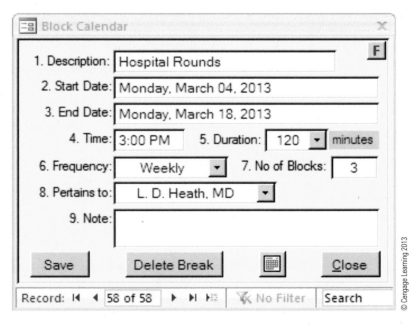

FIGURE 3-2: Completed block calendar screen.

7. Click *OK* through the prompt, and then click *Close* on the Block Calendar window. The time is now blocked off on the Practice Schedule calendar **(see Figure 3-3)**. (To navigate to March 4, use the calendar in the upper-right corner of the screen. Use the Y–/Y+ and M–/M+ buttons to select the correct year and month, and then click on the day within the calendar to bring up the schedule for that date.)

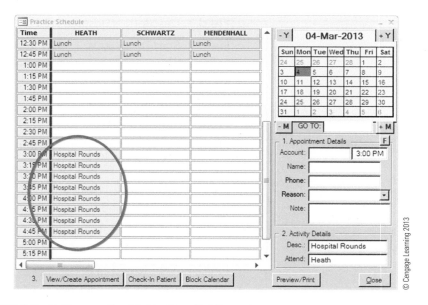

FIGURE 3-3: Setting up the Matrix: Hospital Rounds.

8. Enter the following activities to be blocked in the calendar for Dr. Heath:

   a. Tuesday, March 5, 2013: Staff Breakfast from 9:00 to 10 a.m., one time only.

   b. Tuesday, March 5, 2013: 4:00 p.m. Lecture at Douglasville Community College for 2 hours, weekly for 2 weeks

   c. Thursday, March 7, 2013: Hospital Rounds from 3:30 to 6:00 p.m., one time block

   d. Friday, March 8, 2013: Office Staff Meeting from 4:00 to 6:00 p.m., one time block

9. Now, delete the break for the two lectures at Douglasville Community College for Dr. Heath.

   a. Click *Block Calendar* on the bottom of the Practice Schedule.

   b. Click *Yes* at the prompt.

   c. Use the record locator **(see Figure 3-4)** on the bottom of the Block Calendar window to find the entry you previously created.

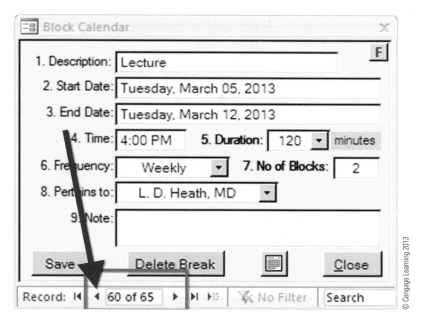

FIGURE 3-4: Scroll through the blocks existing in the program using the record locator arrows.

    d. When you find the correct entry, click *Delete Break*. Click *Yes* through the prompt, and then close to return to the Practice Schedule calendar.

10. Now, create a new break for Tuesday, March 5, 2013: Lecture at Douglasville Community College at 4:00 p.m. for 2 hours, one time only.

JOB 6-2 # PATIENT REGISTRATION AND HIPAA PRIVACY PRACTICES

Patient registration requires that a patient completes the registration forms on or before his or her first visit to the office. Many offices mail information sheets to the patient prior to the first visit to be completed and either have the patient mail the forms back to the office or bring them in at the time of the visit.

Registering New Patients

1. Click *Patient Registration* on the Main Menu to begin to register Margaret Chandler, whose registration information can be found on the ledger card you prepared on March 4 in Section 2, when she came to the office as a new patient (see **Job 1-1**).

2. Even though you know Margaret Chandler is a new patient, it is always a good idea to check that her name is not in the system. In the Patient Registration search window, type a few letters of the patient's last name in the Search Criteria field. Click *Search* (**see Figure 3-5**).

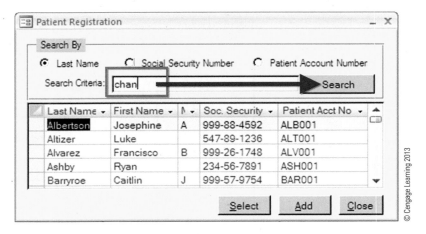

FIGURE 3-5: Search for a patient by typing the first few letters of the last name, and clicking *Search*.

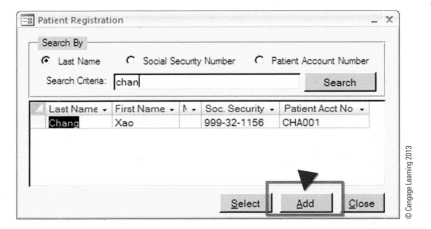

FIGURE 3-6: Use the *Add* button when registering new patients.

3. Her name does not appear, meaning she is not registered in the system. Click *Add* at the bottom of the pop-up screen (**see Figure 3-6**).

4. A blank patient record appears. Complete the Patient Information tab (Fields 1–20) using the information on Margaret Chandler's ledger card. Check your work with **Figure 3-7**. Click *Save*.

5. Working your way across the tabs, click on the Spouse/Parent/Other tab. Complete Fields 1–6. Click *Save*.

6. Click the *Address* icon. If the address is different from the patient's address, it is entered in this section. If the address is the same as the patient's address, click *Copy Pt Addr*. There is no need to complete the lower section in this area. Check your work with **Figure 3-8**. Click *Save*.

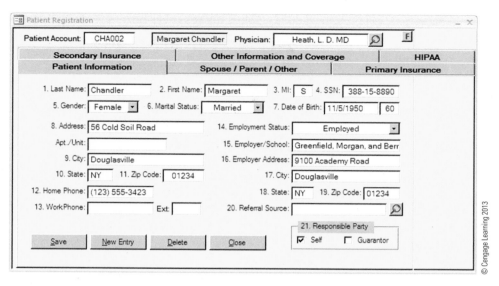

FIGURE 3-7: Completed Patient Information tab for Margaret Chandler.

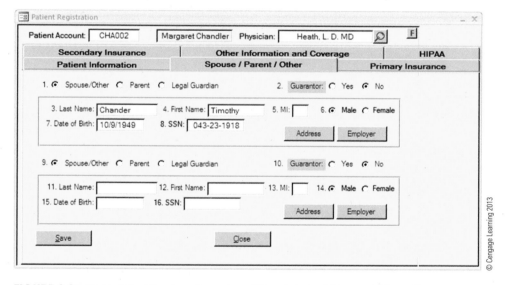

FIGURE 3-8: Completed Spouse, Parent, or Other tab for Margaret Chandler.

7. Click on the Primary Insurance tab and complete Fields 1–16.

    a. In Field 1, click on the magnifying glass icon to bring up a search window. Search for FlexiHealth PPO. Dr. Heath participates with FlexiHealth, so double click the row for FlexiHealth PPO In-Network to select it as the insurance plan for this patient.

    b. In Field 2, select the radio button next to Self. Note that when you do, several fields in the Policyholder Information section autopopulate with data already entered.

    c. Type the insurance ID number in Field 8 and the group number in Field 10. Leave Field 9 blank.

    d. Enter the patient's co-pay amount in Field 12.

e. Select the Yes check boxes in Fields 13–15.

f. Leave Field 16 blank.

8. Check your work with **Figure 3-9**. Click *Save*.

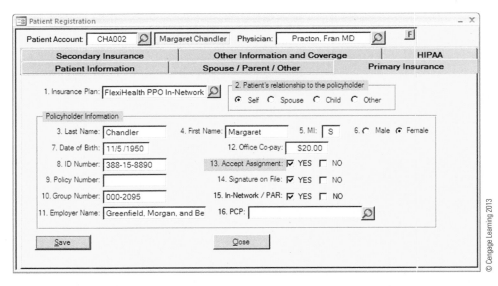

FIGURE 3-9: Completed Primary Insurance tab for Margaret Chandler.

9. There is no need to complete the Secondary Insurance tab because Mrs. Chandler does not have secondary insurance. If a patient has secondary insurance, complete Fields 1–16. Be sure to check the box in Field 11, to Bill Secondary Insurance after Primary. Click *Save*. Remember, it is essential to click *Save* or the information you just entered will not be saved.

10. The Other Information and Coverage tab does not need to be completed because Mrs. Chandler only has a primary insurance carrier. Once again, if you have a patient needing information entered in that tab, complete Fields 1–13. Note that the default in Field 13 (Accident) is *No*, but can be changed if necessary.

11. Click on the last tab, HIPAA. On the ledger card for Mrs. Chandler, you will notice it states that the HIPAA Notice of Privacy Practices was given to the patient and that she signed the acknowledgment of reading and receiving the notice. The Notice of Privacy Practices can be printed out by clicking on the *Privacy Notice* icon on this tab; it is given to new patients at the time of registration or to patients who have not received the notice in the past. A separate form stating that the patient has received and read the form is signed by the patient and kept in the medical record. Check the boxes next to Yes in Fields 1 and 2 and type 03/04/2013 as the date. Leave Field 3 blank.

12. Check your work with **Figure 3-10**. Click *Save*. Click *Close* until you return to the Main Menu.

13. Now, add Pamela Cameron to MOSS as a new patient, using the information from her ledger card (see **Job 1-2**).

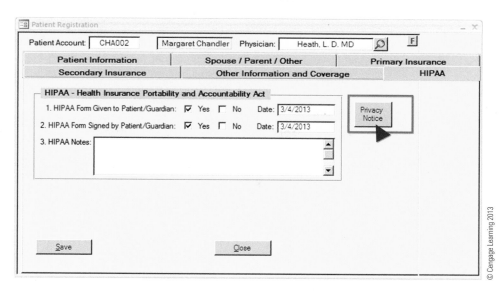

FIGURE 3-10: Completed HIPAA tab for Margaret Chandler.

Updating Established Patients' Medical Records

14. New information needs to be added to Aimee Bradley's medical record. Click on *Patient Registration* in the Main Menu.

15. In the Patient Registration search window, enter the last few letters of the patient's name in the Search Criteria field and click *Search*.

16. When Aimee Bradley appears in the list, you can double-click on her name, or highlight the row, and click *Select* (**see Figure 3-11**).

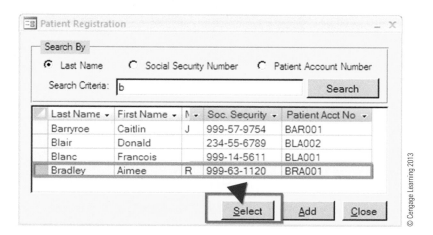

FIGURE 3-11: Searching for established patient Aimee Bradley.

17. On the top bar, note that Aimee's physician is listed as Dr. Schwartz. Click on the magnifying glass icon (**see Figure 3-12**) to change her Physician to Dr. Heath. When the Search Practice Physician window appears, double-click on Dr. Heath's name. Dr. Heath's name is now populated in the Physician field for the patient.

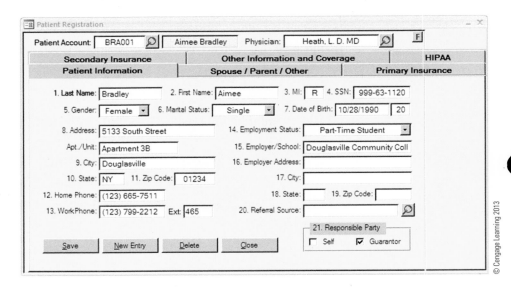

© Cengage Learning 2013

FIGURE 3-12: Change the patient's physician by clicking on the magnifying glass icon on the Patient Registration screen.

18. Additionally, update the following information on the Patient Information tab:
   a. **Field 8.** Add Apartment 3B.
   b. **Field 12.** Update to (123) 665-7511.
   c. **Field 13.** Add (123) 799-2212 Ext 465.
   d. **Field 14.** Change to Part-Time Student.

19. Check your work with **Figure 3-13**. Click *Save*.

© Cengage Learning 2013

FIGURE 3-13: Updated Patient Information tab for Aimee Bradley.

20. Click on the Insurance tab, and update the patient's copayment amount to $15.00. Click *Save*. Close the patient's record when you have finished.

21. Select Isabel Durand's medical record and open the Spouse/Parent/Other tab. Update the following information:
   a. **Field 1.** Change to Legal Guardian.
   b. Add the following information: James A. Durand, 223 Riverside Ave, Douglasville, NY 01234. D.O.B: May 6, 1971; SSN: 225-67-9987; Home Phone: (123) 555-7196
   c. Check your work with **Figure 3-14**. Click *Save*. Close the patient's record when you have finished.

22. Search for and select Megan Caldwell's medical record. On the Patient Information tab, change her physician to Dr. Heath.

23. Search for and select Deanna Hartsfeld's medical record. On the Primary Insurance tab, update her insurance co-pay amount to $15.00.

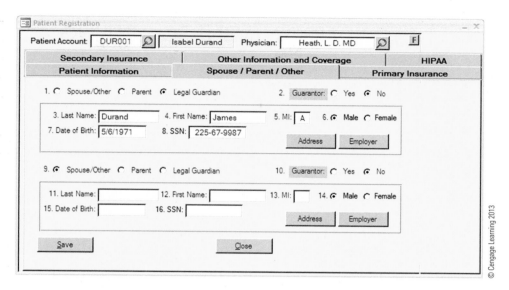

FIGURE 3-14: Updated Spouse/Parent/Other tab for Isabel Durand.

24. Search for and select Nancy Herbert's medical record.

    a. On the Patient Information tab, update her address (Field 8) to 2233 Silver Lane, and zip code (Field 11) to 01234. Update her telephone number (Field 12) to (123) 456-9965.

    b. On the HIPAA tab, update Fields 1 and 2; enter March 4, 2013.

25. Search for and select Xao Chang's medical record.

    a. On the Primary Insurance tab, update his co-pay amount to $15.00.

    b. On the Secondary Insurance tab, update his insurance plan to Century Senior Gap. In Field 1, use the magnifying glass icon to locate the plan name. The ID Number (Field 8) is 99776156 and Group Number (Field 10) is 000-001-223. Leave all other fields the same.

    c. On the HIPAA tab, in Fields 1 and 2, select *Yes* and date March 7, 2013. In Field 3, add to the existing note that Mr. Chang's son was given a copy of the HIPAA regulations.

26. Search for and select Josephine Albertson's medical record. Make the following changes to her account:

    a. Ms. Albertson has moved to 2435 Mt. Vernon Rd, Apartment 3G, Douglasville, NY 01234. Her new home phone number is (123) 665-4465. She got married and will be using a hyphenated name, Albertson-Smith; Field 6 (Marital Status) also needs to be changed.

    b. Complete Fields 1–6 in the Spouse/Parent/Other tab with the following information: Walter P. Smith; D.O.B. 12/12/1948; SSN: 330-26-3321; he is not the guarantor. All the other information stays the same.

27. Search for and select Andrew Jefferson's medical record.

    a. Change his physician to Dr. Heath on the Patient Information tab.

    b. He signs and is given a copy of the office's Notice of Privacy of Practices at his appointment on March 8, 2013. Update this information on the HIPAA tab.

APPOINTMENT SCHEDULING

Creating New Appointments

1. Click *Appointment Scheduling* from the Main Menu.

2. Navigate to March 7, 2013, on the calendar. On the top-right corner of the Practice Schedule, you can either type 03/07/2013 in the GO TO: field and press Enter on the keyboard **(see Figure 3-15)** or by using the Y–/Y+ and M–/M+ buttons and selecting the date on the calendar **(see Figure 3-16).**

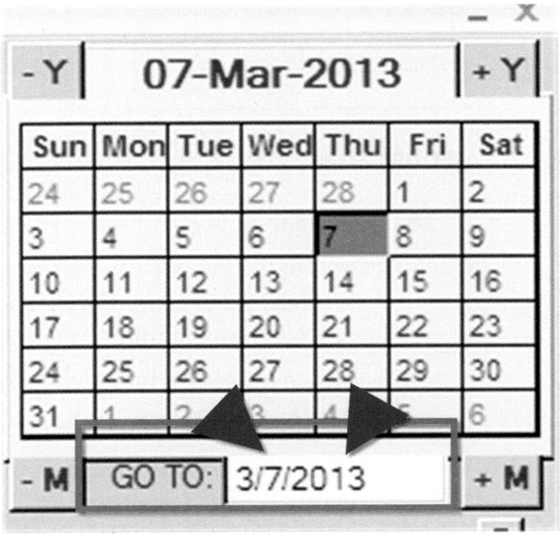

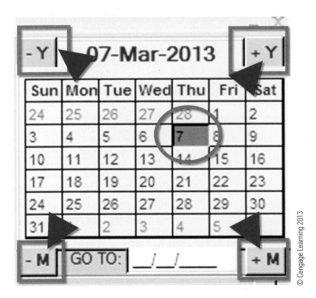

FIGURE 3-15: Type the desired calendar date in the GO TO: field and press Enter on the keyboard.

FIGURE 3-16: Use the Y–/Y+ and M–/M+ to navigate to the desired calendar.

3. Click *View/Create Appointment.*
4. Use the Appointment Scheduling search window to locate Xao Chang and click on *Add*, because you are adding a new appointment for the patient (**see Figure 3-17**).

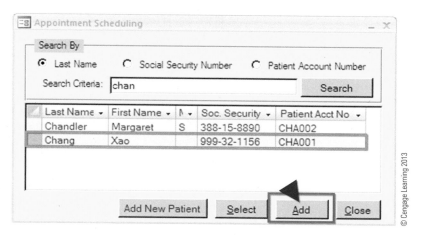

FIGURE 3-17: Search for the patient's name and click *Add.*

5. The Patient Appointment Form window opens. Complete as follows:
   a. **Field 1.** Already completed.
   b. **Field 2.** Use the magnifying glass icon and select Dr. Heath by double-clicking on his name.
   c. **Field 3.** Enter 03/07/2013 (if not already completed).
   d. **Field 4.** Enter 11:00 a.m.
   e. **Field 5.** Select 60 minutes from the drop-down list.
   f. **Field 6.** Select V8 (Special Procedure) from the drop-down list; Mr. Chang will be seen for a complete physical exam.
   g. **Field 7.** Select Single from the drop-down list.
   h. **Field 8.** Autopopulates, leave as is.
   i. **Field 9.** In the Note: field, enter the reason for the visit, which is Complete Physical Exam (other examples might be, sore throat, sneezing, or runny nose). You can leave the rest of the information in Field 9 blank at this time.

6. Check your work with **Figure 3-18**. Click *Save Appointment.*
7. Click *Print* and add the appointment slip to your folder of work to hand in to your instructor. Click *Close* to return to the Practice Schedule. Mr. Chang's appointment now appears on the Practice Schedule.
8. Schedule an appointment for Jordan Connell on Wednesday, March 6, 2013, at 2:30 p.m. for a Complete Physical Exam. Allow 45 minutes and enter V8 (Special Procedure) in Field 6 *Reason,* for a one-time visit. Print an appointment slip and add to your folder of work.

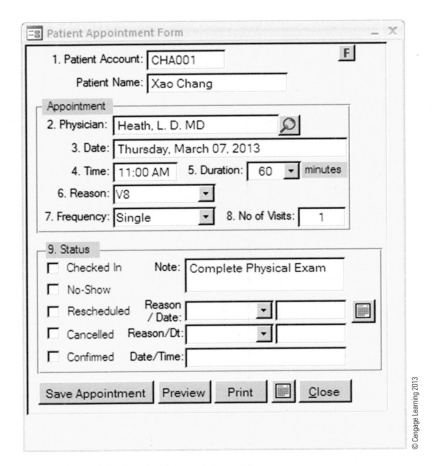

© Cengage Learning 2013

FIGURE 3-18: Completed patient appointment form.

9. Schedule an appointment for Megan Caldwell on Monday, March 11, 2013, at 9:00 a.m. She requires an office visit (15 minutes) for a urinary tract infection.

10. Schedule an appointment for Nancy Herbert on Wednesday, March 6, 2013, at 3:15 p.m.; she requires a recheck (Office Visit, 15 minutes) for a UTI.

11. Schedule an appointment for Aimee Bradley on Tuesday, March 5, 2013, at 3:30 p.m. for an office visit (15 minutes). She is complaining of red, watery eyes.

12. Schedule an appointment for Josephine Albertson-Smith on Monday, March 11, 2013, at 1:00 p.m. for an office visit (15 minutes). She would like to see the doctor because she has a sore throat.

13. Schedule an appointment for Cynthia Worthington on Monday, March 11, 2013, at 1:15 p.m. for an office visit (15 minutes). She states she has an earache.

● ## "No-Shows"

14. Aimee Bradley is scheduled for 3:30 p.m. on Tuesday, March 5, 2013, but never arrived for her appointment (see **Job 2-16**). Find Ms. Bradley's appointment on the Practice Schedule on Tuesday, March 5. (Use the calendar in the upper-right corner to navigate to the date.)

15. Double-click on the appointment on the Practice Schedule.

16. The Patient Appointment Form appears. In Field 9 (Status), check *No Show* (**see Figure 3-19**).

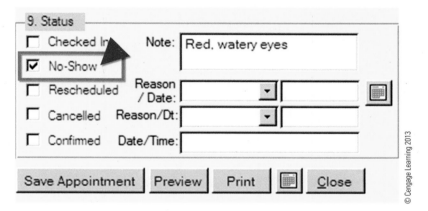

FIGURE 3-19: Updating the appointment Status field for a no-show patient.

17. Click *Save Appointment*.

18. Aimee Bradley calls early on Wednesday, March 6, 2013, and apologizes for missing her appointment yesterday and asks if she can be seen this morning (see **Job 3-1**). Schedule a new appointment for her at 10:00 a.m. Print an appointment slip and add to your folder of work.

Rescheduling Appointments

19. Nancy Herbert calls to reschedule her March 6, 2013, at 3:15 p.m. She forgot she has another doctor's appointment at that time. Schedule her for earlier that day, at 11:15 a.m. Find Ms. Herbert's previous appointment on the Practice Schedule on March 6.

20. Double-click on the appointment on the Practice Schedule.

21. The Patient Appointment Form window appears:

   a. In Field 9 (Status), check Rescheduled.

   b. Next to Reason/Date, select R6 (Needs different date) from the drop-down list.

   c. Then, continuing across the row, click the *Rescheduling Calendar* icon **(see Figure 3-20)**.

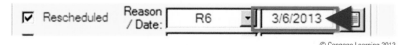

FIGURE 3-20: The Rescheduling Calendar icon.

22. The Practice Reschedule appears *(it looks identical to the Practice Schedule, except the top bar reads Practice Reschedule).* Use the calendar in the upper-right corner to click on Wednesday, March 6, 2013 (if not already selected). Then, double-click on the 11:15 a.m. timeslot **(see Figure 3-21).** *At this point, it will appear that nothing has happened.* In the Appointment Details section on the right side of the screen, 11:15 AM should now be populated.

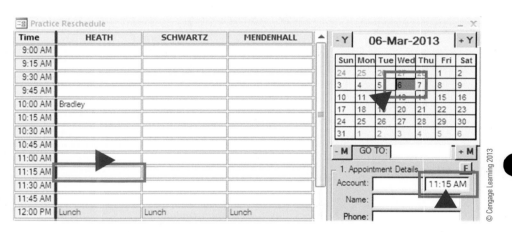

FIGURE 3-21: Use the calendar to navigate to the new desired date, and double-click in the new appointment timeslot.

23. Click *Close* on the bottom-right corner of the Practice Reschedule.

24. Now, the Patient Appointment Form appears again. Note that a date (3/6/2013) appears in Field 9, Rescheduled Date field **(see Figure 3-22).**

FIGURE 3-22: If done correctly, the rescheduled date will appear on the Patient Appointment Form.

25. Click *Save Appointment.* Click *OK* through the prompt.

26. Click *Close* to return to the Practice Schedule. Check the Practice Schedule for March 6 at 11:15 a.m. to verify Ms. Herbert's rescheduled appointment.

27. Now, reschedule Megan Caldwell's appointment (originally on Monday, March 11), for Friday, March 8, 2013, at 9:15 a.m. Her symptoms are more severe and she would like to be seen sooner.

Appointment Cancellations

28. Josephine Albertson-Smith has an appointment scheduled for March 11. She calls on Thursday, March 7, and says she is feeling fine now and doesn't need to be seen. Go to the appointment date on the Practice Schedule and double-click on the patient's name. The Patient Appointment Form appears.

29. In Field 9, select the box next to the option that applies, in this case, Cancelled.

30. Continuing across the row, use the drop-down menu to select the reason for the cancellation (C2—Feeling Fine Now), and then type the date the appointment was cancelled (March 7, 2013).

31. Check your work with **Figure 3-23** and then click *Save Appointment*. Click *OK* through the confirming prompts. Click *Close*, and note that the appointment no longer appears on the Practice Schedule.

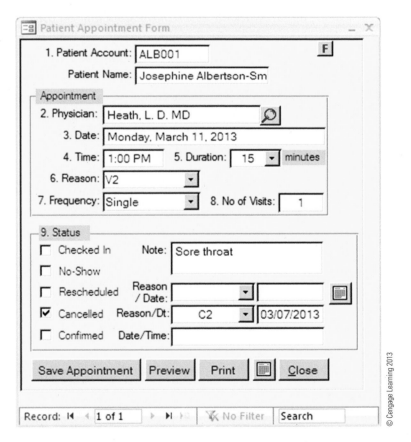

FIGURE 3-23: Cancelling a patient's appointment.

32. Cynthia Worthington calls the office on Friday, March 8, 2013. She doesn't have a ride to her office visit on Monday, so she has to cancel the appointment. She will call back for an appointment when she is able to get a ride.

JOB 6-4 PATIENT CHECK-IN

Patient check-in is the time to review any information that may have changed since the patient's last visit. It is always a good idea to ask the patient for his or her insurance ID card and to make a copy of both sides of the card because many times some information may have changed that the patient may not be aware of. For example, the patient may have the same insurance carrier, the same identification number, but perhaps the co-pay amount changed, or the group number may have changed. If the patient's address changed it is important that the insurance carrier knows about this change. Not having the correct information could cause an insurance claim to be denied. Since most insurance carriers now allow between 90 to 120 days for a claim to be processed, it is important for the front office professional to be diligent on collecting the most up-to-date information about a patient.

Schedule Check-In

1. Click on *Appointment Scheduling* on the Main Menu. Aimee Bradley arrives for her appointment on March 6, 2013.

2. Select the date needed, using the calendar in the upper-right corner of the Practice Schedule screen.

3. Find the patient's name on the Practice Schedule. Click once on the patient's name, and notice that the appointment information for the patient appears in the Appointment Detail box on the right side of the screen, under the calendar.

4. Check *Check-In* on the bottom of the screen (**see Figure 3-24**); this records that the patient has checked in. Click *OK* through the prompt, confirming the patient is marked as checked in. Click *Close* to return to the Main Menu.

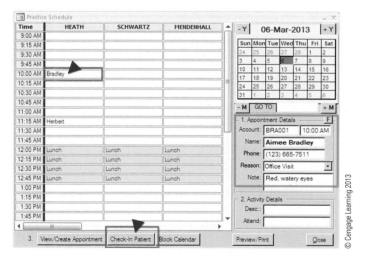

FIGURE 3-24: Checking in a patient on the Practice Schedule.

5. Nancy Herbert arrives for her appointment on March 6, 2013. Indicate on the appointment schedule that she has checked in.

6. Jordan Connell arrives for his appointment on March 6, 2013. Indicate on the appointment schedule that he has checked in.

Online Insurance Eligibility

Many offices have the ability to use an online eligibility function of the computer system to check the status of the patient's insurance. Most insurance identification cards list the date that the insurance became effective but they don't list the expiration date. In the pegboard system, a Point-of Service (POS) device was used to verify if the patient's insurance was current prior to the visit with the physician. A computer system program has the ability to verify a patient's current insurance by processing it through the online eligibility function provided on the computer program.

1. On the Main Menu, click *Online Eligibility*.

2. Search for Aimee Bradley in the Online Eligibility search window, and click *Select* to pull up her insurance information.

3. Verify that the information listed matches the information on her present insurance card, and click *Send to Payer* (see **Figure 3-25**).

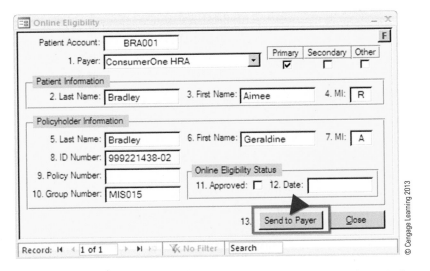

FIGURE 3-25: Verify that all information is correct on the Online Eligibility window.

4. When the online eligibility status completes, click on *View* (see **Figure 3-26**).

5. Click *Print* to print out a copy of the Online Eligibility Transmission Report and place it in the patient's medical record. In this simulation, print the form and add it to your folder of work to hand in to your instructor. Click *Close* to return to the Main Menu.

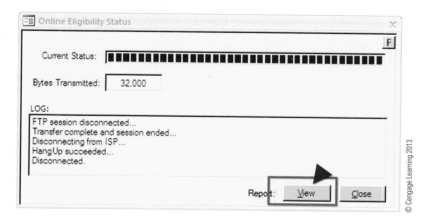

FIGURE 3-26: Completed Online Eligibility Status window.

6. Verify new patient Margaret Chandler's insurance information using the Online Eligibility function of MOSS. Print out a copy of the Online Eligibility Transmission Report and add it to your folder of work.

7. Verify new patient Pamela Cameron's insurance information using the Online Eligibility function of MOSS. Print out a copy of the Online Eligibility Transmission Report and add it to your folder of work.

8. Verify Nancy Herbert's insurance information using the Online Eligibility function of MOSS. Print out a copy of the Online Eligibility Transmission Report and add it to your folder of work.

9. Verify Jordan Connell's insurance information using the Online Eligibility function of MOSS. Print out a copy of the Online Eligibility Transmission Report and add it to your folder of work.

JOB 6-5 · POSTING CHARGES

Accurate financial transactions and records are essential to the efficient running of a medical office, whether the transaction is done by a pegboard system or a computer system. The medical office professional has the legal and ethical responsibility to be accurate with coding and charges. Now that you are familiar with locating patient information in the computer system, you will now be asked to post charges, payments, adjustments, process refunds, NSF, and payments from collection agencies, all skills learned in the first part of this simulation. Let's begin with posting charges.

Office Charges

Posting charges and payments in MOSS requires two different procedures, unlike the pegboard system where the entire transaction of charges, adjustments, and payment can be made at the same time.

1. To begin, click *Procedure Posting* from the Main Menu. Aimee Bradley was seen in the office on March 6, 2013 (Level 2 Office Visit), and was diagnosed with conjunctivitis (see **Job 3-4**).

2. Search for Aimee Bradley's name in the Procedure Posting search window. Click *Add* (**see Figure 3-27**), because you are going to add procedures to the patient's account.

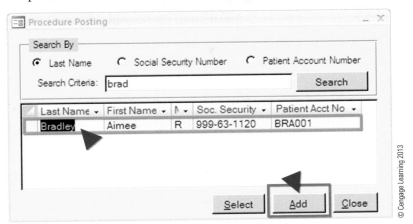

FIGURE 3-27: Locate the patient's account, and click *Add* to post new procedures.

3. The Procedure Posting window appears. Fill in the following fields:

   a. **Field 1.** Type 111. The posting entry will not be able to be processed without a reference number. For this simulation, you will add the reference number 111 to all posting procedures.

   b. **Field 2.** Automatically fills in with the patient's doctor selected in Patient Registration; in this case, Dr. Heath. Do not change this.

   c. **Field 3.** Select office (11) from the drop-down list, because the patient was seen in the office.

   d. **Field 4.** Leave blank. This field is used only if the patient was seen at a facility other than the office, such as a hospital or skilled nursing facility.

   e. **Field 5.** Type 03/06/2013 for the date of service (DOS), the date the patient was treated.

   f. **Field 6.** Leave blank. These fields are used only if the service was performed over multiple days, for example, when posting hospital charges.

   g. **Field 7.** Automatically fills in based on Fields 5 and 6. A "1" will be displayed if the patient was seen in the office.

   h. **Field 8.** Click on the magnifying glass icon and select *99212*, the CPT code for Aimee Bradley's office visit.

   i. **Field 9.** Leave blank for Aimee Bradley. If a modifier was required, you would use the drop-down list to select the appropriate modifier.

   j. **Field 10.** Automatically fills in based on Fields 8 and 9.

   k. **Field 11.** Automatically fills in based on the patient's insurance selected in Patient Registration.

   l. **Field 12.** Use the magnifying glass icon to search and select the appropriate ICD code (Conjunctivitis, Unspec., 372.30).

Up to four diagnoses can be entered per insurance claim using letters a–d.

m. **Field 13.** Leave this as the default, which is *no*.

4. Compare your entries with **Figure 3-28** to ensure all fields are correct.

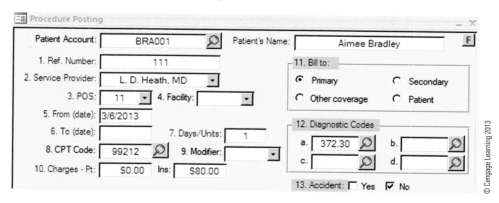

FIGURE 3-28: Entering procedure charges for Aimee Bradley.

5. Click *Post* at the bottom of the Procedure Posting window.

6. Note that when you click *Post*, the procedure charge entered at the top of the screen now appears in the Posting Detail area, in the middle of the screen (**see Figure 3-29**). Additionally, the information is entered in the Summary of Charges in Field 15.

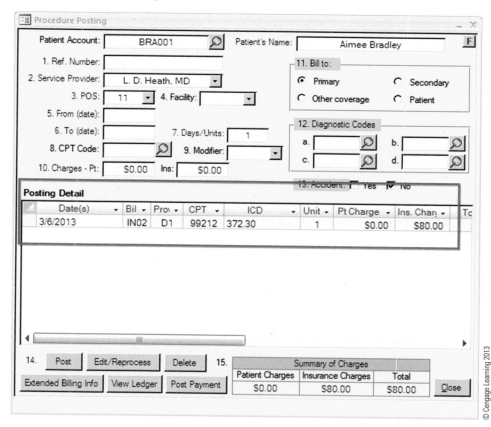

FIGURE 3-29: Once procedure charges are posted, they appear in the Posting Detail area.

7. If you needed to enter more procedures, you would go back to the top section of the Procedure Posting window (Fields 1–13) and enter the next procedure, clicking *Post* after each completed entry. In this case, there are no additional procedures to post.

8. When all charges have been entered, click *Close*, located at the bottom right of the screen, until you return to the Main Menu.

Correcting an Error in Procedure Posting

> Errors happen when posting and can be corrected by following these steps:
>
> a. In the Posting Detail section, highlight the row of the charge that contains the error.
>
> b. Click *Edit/Reprocess*.
>
> c. You will notice that the entire entry is removed from Posting Detail but has reappeared in Fields 1–13, which allows it to be edited.
>
> d. Re-enter the correct information in Fields 1–13. Double-check your work for accuracy.
>
> e. Click *Post* when completed. The charge now appears back in the Posting Detail section.

9. Post the following charges for Nancy Herbert's office visit on 3/6/2013 (see **Job 3-7**): Level 3 Office Visit, urine (81000), and blood sugar (82947). Diagnoses: diabetes mellitus, type II controlled, and urinary tract infection, unspec. When entering the blood sugar procedure, only use the ICD code for diabetes mellitus; when entering the UA/routine with microscopy, only use the ICD code for UTI. (Recall that you will use reference number 111 for all procedure postings.) Check your work with **Figure 3-30**.

Posting Detail

Date(s)	Bil	Pro	CPT	ICD	Unit	Pt Charge	Ins. Char	Tc
3/6/2013	IN04	D1	99213	250.00 + 599.0	1	$0.00	$111.00	S
3/6/2013	IN04	D1	81000	250.00	1	$0.00	$12.00	
3/6/2013	IN04	D1	82947	599.0	1	$0.00	$19.00	

FIGURE 3-30: Completed Posting Detail for Nancy Herbert.

© Cengage Learning 2013

10. Post the charges for Margaret Chandler for her 3/4/2013 office visit (see **Job 1-1**).

11. Post the charges for Pamela Cameron for her 3/4/2013 office visit (see **Job 1-2**).

12. Post the charges for Xao Chang for his 3/7/2013 office visit (see **Job 4-6**).

13. Post the charges for Deanna Hartsfeld for her 3/7/2013 office visit (see **Job 4-9**). The diagnoses are headaches and hypertension, unspec.

14. Post the charges for Megan Caldwell for her 3/8/2013 office visit (see **Job 5-2**).

15. Post the charges for Andrew Jefferson for his 3/8/2013 office visit (see **Job 5-5**).

Hospital Charges

Posting hospital charges follows similar steps, with a few modifications. Post Isabel Durand's charges from January 26–30, 2013, at Community General Hospital (see **Job 3-5**).

16. Begin by clicking *Procedure Posting* from the Main Menu.

17. Search for Isabel Durand in the patient list. Select her name, and click *Add*, to add new charges to her account.

18. Post the first charge, the hospital admission (99221). Complete the Procedure Posting window as follows for this charge:

    a. **Field 1.** 111.

    b. **Field 2.** Already populated with the patient's doctor (Dr. Heath).

    c. **Field 3.** Select Inpatient (21) from the drop-down list.

    d. **Field 4.** Select Community General Hospital (F2) from the drop-down list.

    e. **Field 5.** Enter the admission date 1/26/2013.

    f. **Field 6.** Leave blank, because the one-day admission date was entered in Field 5. If you enter the hospital admission date in Field 5 and the hospital discharge date in Field 6, the charge for the hospitalization will not be correct due to different CPT codes for admission, subsequent visits, and discharge; recall that each has its own different charge amount.

    g. **Field 7.** Automatically fills in with the number 1 (this field auto-populates based on Fields 5 and 6).

    h. **Field 8.** Type 99221 (CPT code for hospital admission). You can also use the magnifying glass icon to search and select the code.

    i. **Field 9.** Leave blank; there is no modifier necessary.

    j. **Fields 10** and **11.** Automatically fills in from the fee schedule within the program when you select the CPT code.

    k. **Field 12.** Type 496 (the ICD code for COPD); this field can have up to four diagnoses, if applicable.

    l. **Field 13.** Leave as the default answer of *No*, because the hospitalization was not due to an accident.

19. Review your entries to ensure accuracy. Click *Post*. The charge should now appear in the Posting Detail section.

20. Next, you will continue posting the hospital daily charges for the dates 1/27 to 1/30/2013, four daily visits. Adding daily charges are similar to adding additional office procedures. Go back up to Field 1, and follow the above steps until you get to:

    a. **Field 5.** Type 1/27/2013 (the first daily hospital visit).

    b. **Field 6.** Type 1/30/2013 (the last daily hospital visit before the discharge date).

c. **Field 7.** The program automatically calculates 4, based on the From: and To: fields, for four daily hospital visits.

d. **Field 8.** Type 99231 (the CPT code for hospital subsequent care) for the daily hospital visits.

e. **Field 12.** Type 496 (the ICD code for COPD).

f. Check your work with **Figure 3-31**.

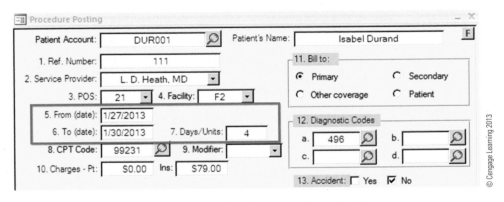

FIGURE 3-31: Procedure Posting entry for subsequent hospital charges.

21. Click *Post*. You will notice that the daily hospital charges 1/27 to 1/30/2013 are now entered in the Posting Detail section, along with the 1/26/2013 hospital admission charge. Scroll over to see the total charge of $316.00 **(see Figure 3-32)**.

Posting Detail

Date(s)	Bil	Prov	CPT	ICD	Unit	Pt Charge	Ins. Char	Total
1/26/2013	IN04	D1	99221	496	1	$0.00	$145.00	$145.00
1/27/2013 to 1/30/2(	IN04	D1	99231	496	4	$0.00	$79.00	$316.00

© Cengage Learning 2013

FIGURE 3-32: Total charges for the daily hospital charges: $79.00 × 4 visits =$316.00.

22. The last charge to enter is the discharge date. Go back up to Field 1, and proceed as before, but in Field 5 enter 1/31/2013 (nothing in Field 6). Enter the discharge CPT code 99238 (hospital discharge services) in Field 8. Complete all the appropriate fields and click *Post*. The last charge has been added to the Procedure Detail section, showing the entire charges for the entire hospital visit. Review the Summary of Charges to see the total charge of $606.00, the same charge amount you entered in the pegboard system **(see Figure 3-33)**.

23. Click *Close* until you return to the Main Menu.

24. Now, post the charge for Isabel Durand for the March 7, 2013, initial hospital admission (see **Job 4-13**).

At this point, we recommend creating a backup file to save your MOSS work up to this point. Please follow the directions on page 150 in Section 4: MOSS Setup and Installation to create a backup file.

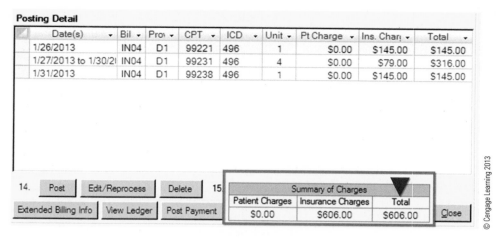

Posting Detail

Date(s) ▾	Bil ▾	Prov ▾	CPT ▾	ICD ▾	Unit ▾	Pt Charge ▾	Ins. Char ▾	Total ▾
1/26/2013	IN04	D1	99221	496	1	$0.00	$145.00	$145.00
1/27/2013 to 1/30/2(	IN04	D1	99231	496	4	$0.00	$79.00	$316.00
1/31/2013	IN04	D1	99238	496	1	$0.00	$145.00	$145.00

14. Post   Edit/Reprocess   Delete   15.

Extended Billing Info   View Ledger   Post Payment

Summary of Charges		
Patient Charges	Insurance Charges	Total
$0.00	$606.00	$606.00

Close

FIGURE 3-33: Posting hospital charges for Isabel Durand.

JOB 6-6 — POSTING PAYMENTS FROM PATIENTS AND INSURANCE PLANS

Payments come from many sources in a medical office. Patients may pay by cash, check, or even credit or debit cards. Checks from insurance carriers are also a form of payment for the physician's services. Posting payments sometimes means making adjustments in the amount of the payment in relation to the charge. Adjustments can be income that will never be collected can be due to a contract agreement the physician makes with the insurance carrier or due to the services of a collection agency, in cases where the physician is having difficulty collecting an outstanding balance from a patient. Payments from collection agencies are handled the same as any other adjustment. A statement from the collection agency will show the amount collected from the patient, the portion owed to the collection agency, and a check for the physician's portion of the money collected by the collection agency. The difference between what was collected and the portion designated to the collection agency must be written off as an adjustment.

Patient Payments

1. Select *Posting Payment* from the Main Menu. Follow these steps to enter Aimee Bradley's $15.00 copayment for her 3/6/13 office visit (see **Job 3-4**).

2. Search for and select the patient's name, Aimee Bradley, and click *Apply Payment.*

3. In MOSS, each payment is posted against a specific charge. Note the top of the Posting Payment window is the Procedure Charge History section. Within this section, click on the row for the appropriate charge (99212) to select it **(see Figure 3-34)**.

4. Click *Select/Edit* (at the bottom of the screen). If done correctly, the balance for that charge will display in Field 13 **(see Figure 3-35)**.

If the Balance Due field does not show the charge amount, do not proceed. Aimee Bradley owes $80.00 for the 99212 office visit on 3/6/2013. If you have performed this step correctly, the $80.00 amount appears in Field 13.

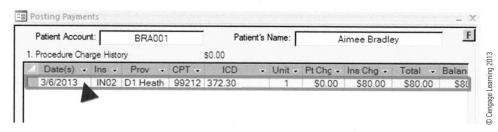

FIGURE 3-34: First, select the charge against which the payment will be posted.

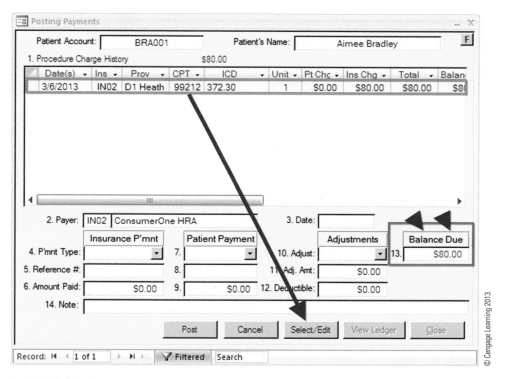

FIGURE 3-35: Highlight the appropriate charge, and click *Select/Edit* to prepare to post a payment against the charge.

5. Now, complete the following fields:
   a. **Field 2.** Leave as is; this automatically shows the patient's insurance.
   b. **Field 3.** Type 3/6/2013 (the same date as the procedure charge).
   c. **Field 4-6.** Skip these fields, as they are used to record insurance payments. If the payment is made by the patient, only Fields 7–9 are used.

    d. **Field 7.** Select PATCASH from the drop-down list. This field allows you to select payment types of *Cash, Check, or Other. Other* refers to a credit or debit card the patient may use.

    e. **Field 8.** This is used when *Other* is selected as the payment type in Field 7, and would be used to enter the type of credit or debit card used for payment. In this case, since the patient paid with cash, leave blank.

    f. **Field 9.** Type $15.00, the amount the patient paid.

    g. **Fields 10-12.** Skip these fields; they are used when recording Adjustments and Deductibles.

    h. **Field 14.** Leave blank. This field can be used to record other information about the payment.

6. Check your work with **Figure 3-36**. **MOSS does not allow corrections to payments, once posted, so review your entries carefully.**

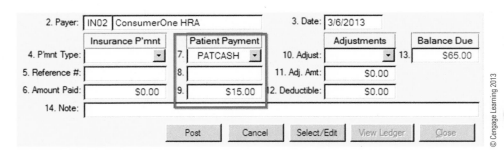

FIGURE 3-36: Patient copayment posting for Aimee Bradley's office visit charge.

7. Click *Post* at the bottom of the screen.

8. To view your posting and the payments made on the patient account, click on *View Ledger.* The Patient Ledger window shows the charges and payments made. Below the Activity portion of the screen (Field 7), use the scroll bar (shown in **Figure 3-37**) and scroll to the right side to see the balance due for each charge.

10. Click *Close* to return to the Posting Payments window. Click *Close* until you return to the Main Menu.

11. Post Margaret Chandler's $20 cash co-pay for her 3/4/2013 office visit (99202) (see **Job 1-1**).

12. Post Xao Chang's $15 cash co-pay for his 3/7/2013 visit. Be sure to post against the correct procedure, the well-adult exam (99397) (see **Job 4-6**).

13. Post Deanna Hartsfeld's $15 cash co-pay for her 3/7/2013 office visit (99213) (see **Job 4-9**).

14. Post Andrew Jefferson's $20 cash co-pay for his 3/8/2013 office visit (99213) (see **Job 5-5**). Be sure to post against the correct visit date.

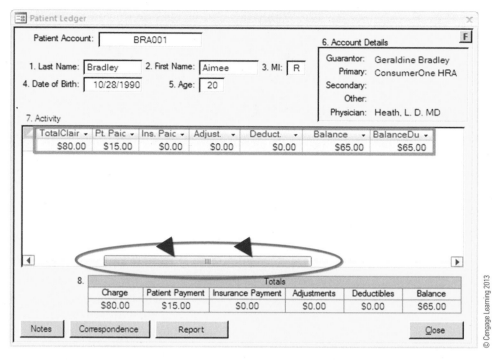

FIGURE 3-37: Use the scroll bar to view the transactions for each procedure charge.

Insurance Payments

15. Select *Posting Payment* from the Main Menu. Follow these steps to complete the payment for Nancy Herbert's 3/6/13 office visit (see **Job 5-15**). A check came from Medicare Statewide Corp. in the amount of $99.25; the insurance adjustment was $32.75 and the $10.00 balance will be billed to Mrs. Herbert. We will be posting a total of three payments, according to the payment breakdown in the Explanation of Benefits that accompanied the check in **Figure 3-38**.

16. Search for and select the patient's name, Nancy Herbert, and click *Apply Payment.*

					MEDICARE- STATEWIDE CORP		
Member's Name	**DOS**	**Units**	**Procedure Code**	**Billed**	**Allowed**	**Member Responsibility**	**Paid to Physician**
Nancy Herbert	3/6	1	99213	111.00	84.45	10.00	74.45
	3/6	1	81000	12.00	9.60	0.00	9.60
	3/6	1	82947	19.00	15.20	0.00	15.20
TOTALS				**142.00**	**32.75**	**10.00**	**99.25**

FIGURE 3-38: Explanation of Benefits for Nancy Herbert.

17. Within this section, click on the row for the first charge (99213) to select it, and then click *Select/Edit*. If done correctly, the balance for that charge ($111.00) will display in Field 13.

18. Now, complete the following fields:

    a. **Field 2.** Leave as is; this automatically shows the patient's insurance.

    b. **Field 3.** Type 3/8/2013 (the date of payment posting).

    c. **Field 4.** Select PAYINS (Payment Insurance) from the drop-down menu, because this is an insurance payment.

    d. **Field 5.** Leave blank.

    e. **Field 6.** Type 74.45, which is the amount the insurance has paid for this charge.

    f. **Fields 7–9.** Skip; these are used when recording a payment from the patient.

    g. **Field 10.** Select ADJINS (Adjustment Insurance) from the drop-down menu; recall from the EOB that the insurance has allowed $84.45, and the remaining amount must be written off as an insurance adjustment.

    h. **Field 11.** Type $26.55, the amount of the adjustment (charges less the allowed amount, $111.00 − $84.45 = $26.55).

    i. **Field 12.** If the patient had a deductible amount, it would be entered here. Mrs. Herbert does not, so leave this field blank.

    j. **Field 14.** Leave blank.

    k. Check your work with **Figure 3-39**. Review your entries carefully. **Remember that MOSS does not allow corrections to payments, so please make your entries carefully and double-check your work.**

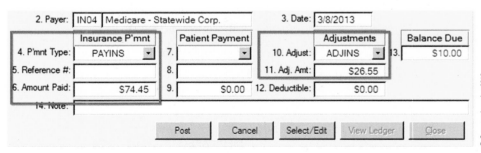

FIGURE 3-39: Insurance payment and adjustment for Nancy Herbert's office visit charge (99213).

19. Click *Post* at the bottom of the screen.

20. Now, post the insurance's payment against the second charge (81000). In the Procedure Charge History area, highlight the charge and click *Select/Edit* at the bottom of the screen **(Figure 3-40)**. If this is done correctly, the Balance Due field will show $12.00.

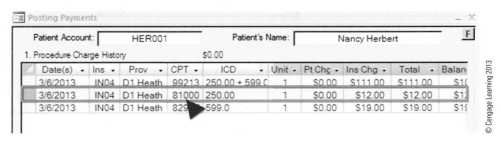

FIGURE 3-40: Select the appropriate charge from the Procedure Charge History area (81000), and then click *Select/Edit.*

21. Fill in the remaining fields with the information from the patient's EOB, using the steps you learned above. Check your work with **Figure 3-41**. Click *Post* to record the payment.

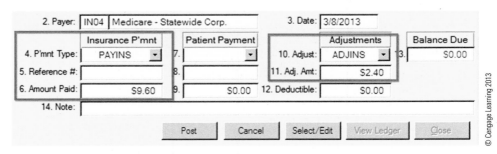

FIGURE 3-41: Insurance payment and adjustment for Nancy Herbert's urine test (81000).

22. Post the insurance's payment against the third charge (82947).

23. To view your posting and the payments made on the patient account, click on *View Ledger.* The Patient Ledger window shows the charges and payments made, and should match the EOB amounts (**see Figure 3-42**). Below the Activity portion of the screen (Field 7), use the scroll bar to see the balance due for each charge.

24. Click *Close* to return to the Posting Payments window; continue to click *Close* until you return to the Main Menu.

JOB 6-7 | POSTING ADJUSTMENTS

Posting Refunds

1. Select *Posting Payments* from the Main Menu. Josephine Albertson-Smith paid a $20.00 copayment for an appointment on July 10, 2009. However, her insurance company did not require a co-pay, and paid the entire procedure charge. She is now entitled to a $20.00 refund.

2. Search for Josephine Albertson-Smith's name in the Posting Payments search window, and click *Apply Payment.*

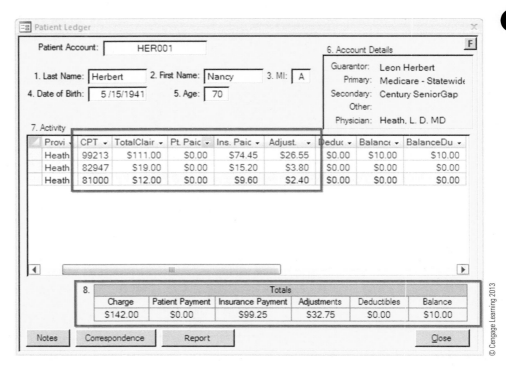

FIGURE 3-42: Nancy Herbert's Patient Ledger, after all insurance payments have been posted.

3. Highlight the procedure row containing the overpayment, CPT code 99212, and click *Select/Edit,* as you have done previously to apply payments. Note: If done properly, the Balance Due field should read ($20.00).

4. Fill out the following fields:

   a. **Field 3.** Overwrite this field with March 4, 2013.

   b. **Field 10.** Select REFUND from the drop-down menu.

   c. **Field 11.** Enter the amount of the refund, $20.00.

   d. Check your work with **Figure 3-43**.

5. Click *Post.* Click *Close* until you return to the Main Menu.

6. Now post a refund for Andrew Jefferson, for $20.00 overpayment of his 7/1/2009 office visit. Use March 4, 2013, as the date of payment posting.

Posting NSF Checks

1. Select *Posting Payments* from the Main Menu. Cynthia Worthington paid a $20.00 copayment with check number 443 for her October 19, 2009,

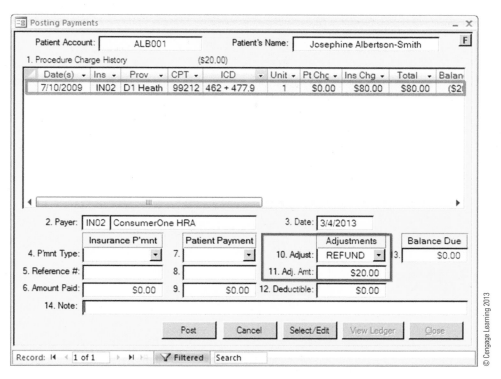

FIGURE 3-43: Posting a refund for Josephine Albertson-Smith.

office visit. The bank notified the office that the account had nonsufficient funds (NSF).

2. Search for Cynthia Worthington's name in the Posting Payments search window, and click *Apply Payment.*

3. Highlight the procedure row containing the overpayment, 10/19/2009 with CPT code 99214, and click *Select/Edit,* as you have done previously to apply payments. Note: If done properly, the Balance Due field should read $0.00.

4. Enter the following information:

   a. **Field 3.** Type 3/4/2013 (you may need to overwrite the date).

   b. **Field 7.** Select OTHER from the drop-down menu.

   c. **Field 8.** Type number 443, the returned check number.

   d. **Field 9.** Type (20.00), the amount of the NSF. The parentheses indicate a negative balance.

   e. **Field 14.** Type "Check #443 returned as NSF".

   f. Check your work with **Figure 3-44**. Note the balance is now $20.00 for this charge.

5. Click *Post.* Click *Close* until you return to the Main Menu.

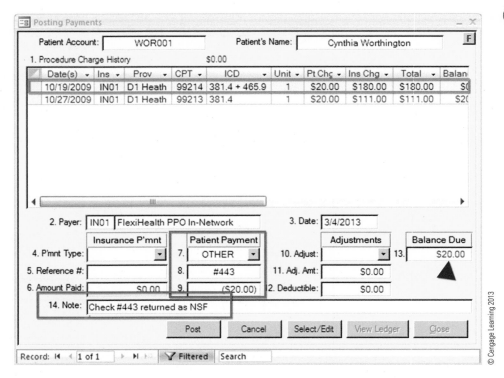

FIGURE 3-44: Posting an NSF for Cynthia Worthington.

JOB 6-8 | PREPARING INSURANCE CLAIMS

Claims are commonly sent electronically through the use of a clearinghouse rather than the tedious task of writing each claim out by hand. Electronic submission of claims has many advantages such as ease of submission because all the information needed has been gathered and entered into the computer system through registration of the patient information, the posting of the charges, and the faster turn-around time from submission of the claims to payment, with some insurance carriers paying within 7 to 10 days. Each office determines the frequency of submitting insurance claims. As part of your experience, in Dr. Heath's office you will help submit insurance claims.

1. Select *Insurance Billing* from the Main Menu.

2. The Claim Preparation window will appear. In Field 1, select Patient Name from the drop-down menu.

3. Fill out Field 2 as follows:

   a. Bill or Rebill: Select Bill.

   b. Provider: Select Dr. Heath from the Provider drop-down list.

   c. Service Dates: From 3/4/2013, Through 3/8/2013.

   d. Patient Name: Select (All) from the drop-down.

   e. Account Number: Leave blank, because you have selected All.

the right-hand corner of the screen to return to the patient billing window. Click *Close* to return to the Main Menu.

JOB 6-10   PRINTING REPORTS

So far in this simulation using a computer system, you have generated Patient Appointment Slips, Online Eligibility Reports, Insurance Billing Worksheets, Claims Submission Reports, and Patient Statement of Accounts. Other reports available with this software include: Aging Reports, Monthly Summaries, and Billing and Payment Report.

1. Click on *Report Generation* from the Main Menu.

2. The Reports Panel appears. We will be creating a Monthly Summary and Billing and Payment Report for March 2013 (**Figure 3-48**).

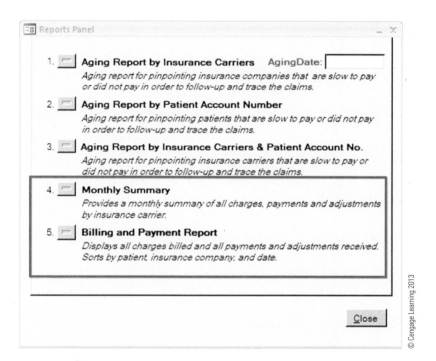

FIGURE 3-48: Reports Panel in MOSS.

3. Click *Monthly Summary*, and use 3/1/2013 as the beginning date and 3/31/2013 as the ending date. Print a copy of this report and put them in your folder to hand in with your work.

4. Go back to the Reports Panel and print out a Billing and Payment Report for March 2013. Print a copy of this report and put them in your folder to hand in with your work.

Your time at Douglasville Medicine Associates is finished. Congratulations! You have successfully completed both sections of this simulation. You have had the experience of processing patient medical records and accounts receivable through a pegboard system and a computer system. Both types of accounting systems are similar and each has its place in a busy, efficient medical front office. As you continue in your chosen profession, may you take with you the knowledge and skills learned in this simulation!

SECTION 4

APPENDIX

Glossary

MOSS Installation and Setup Instructions

Appointment Book Pages

Patient Lists

CMS-1500 Claim Forms

Deposit Slips

Daily Check-up Forms

Section 2 Weekly Check-up

Section 3 Weekly Check-up

GLOSSARY

accept assignment	physician accepts the amount allowed by the insurance plan for payment and will not require the patient to pay the difference
accounts payable	balance due to creditors for supplies and services purchased by the physician
accounts receivable	total balance due from patients for services rendered by the physician
adjustment	amounts of money written off by the physician that consist of the difference between the amount charged by the physician for the procedure and the amount allowed for the procedure by a government insurance program such as Medicare or Medicaid
assignment of benefits	written authorization by the patient giving the insurance company permission to pay the physician directly for services rendered
balance (due)	amount of money owed by a patient to the physician for services rendered
bank balance	amount of money available in a bank account at a given time
beneficiary	person covered under an insurance policy
birthday rule	insurance term for determining primary insurance coverage for children of married parents, both working. The insurance of the parent whose birthday comes first in the year is considered primary.
blank endorsement	has a signature only on the back of a check which allows anyone who signs the check to cash it
Blue Cross	major nonprofit third-party insurance carrier for hospital charges
Blue Shield	major nonprofit third-party insurance carrier for physician and outpatient services
capitation	method of payment for health services by which a health group is prepaid a fixed, per capita amount for each patient served, without considering the actual amount of service provided to each patient
CBC	complete blood count; laboratory test of whole blood to measure the concentration of various types of cells; used to determine the infectious and anemic state of a patient
Centers for Disease Control and Prevention (CDC)	federal agency under the Department of Health and Human Services dedicated to disease prevention and control of diseases all over the country, health promotion and education, and injury prevention
Centers for Medicare and Medicaid (CMS)	federal program, formally known as Health Care Financing Administration (HCFA), and within the Department of Health and Human Services, which oversees and administers the Medicare program and the federal portion of the Medicaid program
charges	fees for procedures performed; may be paid at the time of service in part or in full or may be paid at a later time
check endorsement	transferring the rights of a check from one party to another
check register	record of disbursements from and deposits to a bank account
clearinghouse	service provided for a charge where a company looks over the claims checking for errors, before sending them to the carrier for processing
CMS-1500	Centers for Medicare & Medicaid Services (CMS) universal claim form used for charges to be reimbursed by an insurance carrier
co-insurance	arrangement where the insurance carrier and the patient each pay a percentage of the medical charge; 80/20 is a common distribution of the charges
copayment (co-pay)	part of payment for medical services that the patient is required or chooses to pay at the time services are rendered; also referred to as co-pay
CPT	Current Procedural Terminology; a system used to translate procedures and services into numeric form for standardization
CPT modifiers	two-digit numbers used to supplement information or adjust descriptions providing extra details about a procedure or service, or indicating that it was changed in some way due to specific circumstances
credits	amounts of money received from the patient or an insurance carrier and deducted from the balance due

day sheet	daily log of accounts of patients seen on a given day; shows the total of accounts receivable
deductible	yearly amount of money paid out of the patient's pocket before the insurance carrier pays
donut hole	gap during which the patient has to pay the full out of pocket amount for prescriptions before Medicare resumes prescription payment.
E codes	ICD-CM codes used for coding to explain external causes such as injury, poisoning, and adverse reactions
EKG	electrocardiogram, also known as ECG; a tracing representing the heart's electrical activity; often performed routinely to obtain a baseline for future comparison but may also be used to diagnose heart abnormalities
EOB	Explanation of Benefits; a statement that accompanies payment or rejection of insurance claims
fee schedule	fixed sum set for each professional service
guarantor	person or institution responsible for another's debts or expenses; as with parents for their children
Health Maintenance Organization (HMO)	for-profit health organization in a defined geographic region offering health care to participating members, who must select from list of participating physicians to be reimbursed for medical services; member benefits include reduced out-of-pocket costs, minimal co-pays for office visits
hematocrit	laboratory test used to determine the volume percentage of erythrocytes in whole blood
HIPAA	Health Insurance Portability and Accountability Act; federal law that governs the rules and procedures providing privacy and security of a patient's health information
HIV	human immunodeficiency virus; the virus that causes AIDS
HPN	hypertension
ICD-9-CM codes	*International Classification of Diseases, Ninth Revision, Clinical Modification;* numbers that identify physicians' diagnoses
invoice	bill for goods ordered and shipped or services rendered
ledger card	record of patient information, charges, and payments
Managed Care Organization (MCO)	system of health care that provides health insurance while controlling costs
Medicaid	jointly sponsored federal and state health program administered by state governments, which is designed to help low-income individuals
Medicare	government health insurance program to aid elderly (65 and older) and disabled individuals
Medicare Part A	part of Medicare that helps cover hospital expenses, skilled nursing facilities, home health care, and hospice care
Medicare Part B	part of Medicare that helps pay for visits to the physician and other outpatient services such as laboratory tests, radiology services ambulance service, and durable medical equipment such as wheelchairs, walkers, and commodes, but usually does not cover prescription drugs
Medicare Part C	part of Medicare known as Medicare Advantage plans are alternate plans to the original Medicare plan and are offered by approved private insurance carriers
Medicare Part D	prescription drug plan part of Medicare
Medigap	private insurance to supplement Medicare benefits for noncovered services
morbidity rate	incidence of a disease in a specific locality or of all diseases in a population
mortality rate	death rate or ratio of deaths to a specific population in a specified area
National Provider Identification (NPI)	10-digit unique identification number for health care providers; has replaced all health care provider identifiers in use such as UPIN; this number remains with the health care provider regardless of job or location changes; the number does not carry any information about the health care provider and is used for all HIPAA transactions
nonsufficient funds (NSF)	check that has not been cleared by a bank due to inadequate funds to cover the check
packing slip	provides a list of goods shipped only; no bill is included
payee	person to whom a check is written
payer	person on whose bank account a check will be drawn
payment	amounts of money, either in cash or by check, paid to an individual such as the physician by the patient or an insurance carrier

pegboard system	write-it-once bookkeeping system using specifically designed forms which allow an individual to record data on the top form and simultaneously reproducing it on each form lying beneath it; advantage: saves time and errors by writing data once
petty cash	small sum of cash available for minor expenses that occur in an office
Point-of-Service (POS) device	electrical device that provides immediate and direct access to information concerning the patient's eligibility status by using an electronic network that communicates directly from the medical office to the health care plan of the patient
Preferred Provider Organizations (PPOs)	consists of a group of local physicians who joined together and contract with a managed care organization to provide care to patients at an agreed-on fee
Primary Care Physician (PCP)	physician responsible for coordinating and managing a patient's care, a gatekeeper
primary insurance	insurance coverage that provides benefits after a deductible has been paid by the policy holder regardless of any other insurance policies that may be in effect
procedure codes	five-digit numbers that identify procedures performed by the physician; described in the *Physicians' Current Procedural Terminology*
Resource-Based Relative Value Units (RBRVUs)	value scale for managed care used to determine the value of various physicians' labours; a fee schedule to set the payments for Part B Medicare
restrictive endorsement	prevents anyone other than the endorser, the person for whom the check is intended, from cashing the check
software	term for programs that enable computers to function and perform different tasks
statement	record of patient charges and payments
superbill	document that includes information for insurance carriers and the patient's personal records; may be given to the patient at the time of service
triage	method of screening patients to prioritize and determine the urgency of needed medical care
Tricare	health care program offered by the Department of Defense for members of uniformed services both active and retired, their families, and survivors
usual, reasonable, customary	fee typically charged by a physician for a certain procedure; *reasonable* refers to the midrange of fees charged for a particular service; *customary* refers to the average charge for a specific procedure by all physicians practicing the same specialty in a defined geographic and socioeconomic area
UTI	urinary tract infection
V codes	used for coding factors influencing health status and contact with health services
World Health Organization (WHO)	agency of the United Nations that coordinates public health; responsible for the development of ICD-CM codes to keep track of morbidity and mortality rates

MOSS INSTALLATION AND SETUP INSTRUCTIONS

ABOUT MEDICAL OFFICE SIMULATION SOFTWARE (MOSS) 2.0

Medical Office Simulation Software (MOSS) 2.0 is generic practice management software, realistic in its look and functionality, which helps users prepare to work with any commercial software used in medical offices today. With a friendly, highly graphical interface, MOSS allows users to learn the fundamentals of medical office software packages in an educational environment. It is designed to be used with Section 3.

MOSS SUPPORT AND COMPANION SITE

Tutorials, documentation, and software support and additional resources and tutorials can be found on the MOSS Information, Training, and Support site: **www .cengage.com/community/moss**.

For technical support related to MOSS 2.0, please contact Delmar Technical Support, Monday–Friday, from 8:30 a.m. to 6:30 p.m. Eastern Standard Time.
Phone: 1-800-648-7450
E-mail: **Delmar.help@cengage.com**

INSTALLATION AND SETUP INSTRUCTIONS

These are the installation instructions to install the MOSS 2.0 program from the CD in this package:

1. Close all open programs and documents.
2. Place the Medical Office Simulation Software 2.0 CD into your CD-ROM drive.
3. Medical Office Simulation Software 2.0 should begin setup automatically. Follow the on-screen prompts to install MOSS and Microsoft Access Runtime.
4. Click "Next."
5. Click "I Accept" the terms of the license agreement.
6. Click "Next."
7. Click the button next to "TYPICAL" as the setup type.
8. Click "Install."

If MOSS does not begin setup automatically, follow these instructions:

1. Double-click on My Computer.
2. Double-click the Control Panel icon.

3. Double-click Add/Remove Programs.
4. Click the Install button, and follow the prompts as indicated in step 3.

When you finish installing MOSS, it will be accessible through the Start menu:

- Start > Programs > MOSS v2.0

USING MOSS IN MULTIPLE LOCATIONS: USER SCENARIOS

Scenario 1: MOSS Is Used at a Home Computer

Follow the installation instructions to install MOSS 2.0 single user version onto the home computer. Once MOSS is installed, the user logs in with the username "Student1" and default password "Student1." Changing the password is not necessary. All work is saved on the home computer.

Scenario 2: MOSS Is Used in a School Computer Lab

In a school computer lab, the following routine will need to be performed each time MOSS is used:

1. MOSS single user version needs to be installed on each computer in the lab.
2. The first time a user works in the program: At the end of the session, the user needs to create a backup file when he or she leaves that computer. The Backup utility is found in the File Maintenance section of the program (the next section, Getting Started with MOSS, contains step-by-step instructions).
3. That Backup File should be saved onto a flash drive.
4. The next time the user works on MOSS, insert the flash drive and restore the Backup File that was created at the previous session. The Restore utility is also found in the File Maintenance section of the program; step-by-step instructions are provided in the next section.
5. Each user will need to follow this same routine when working in a classroom lab.
6. To summarize: At the end of each session, the user will create a Backup File saving all work accomplished, and at the beginning of each session, the user will restore the most recent Backup File to continue at the spot where he or she left off.

Scenario 3: MOSS Is Used in Both a Home Computer and a School Computer Lab

Users can work at home and at school, provided that MOSS is installed on every computer on which the user will work. The routine is similar to using MOSS in a school computer lab:

1. MOSS single-user version needs to be installed on the user's home computer and on each computer in the lab.

2. The first time a user works in the program: At the end of the session, the user needs to create a Backup File when he or she leaves that computer. The Backup utility is found in the File Maintenance section of the program (the next section, Getting Started with MOSS, contains step-by-step instructions).

3. That Backup File should be saved onto a flash drive.

4. The next time the user works on MOSS, insert the flash drive and restore the Backup File that was created in the previous session. The Restore utility is also found in the File Maintenance section of the program; step-by-step instructions are provided in the next section.

5. Each user will need to follow this same routine when working in a classroom lab.

6. To summarize: At the end of each session, the user will create a Backup File, saving all work accomplished, and at the beginning of each session, the user will restore the most recent Backup File to continue at the spot where he or she left off.

GETTING STARTED WITH MOSS 2.0

Log-on Instructions

1. When MOSS is launched, it brings up a logon window.

2. The default user name and password are already loaded for you. (The default user name and password is "Student1.")

3. Click OK.

4. You are now at the Main Menu screen of MOSS.

Navigating within the Program

The Main Menu screen orients you to the general functions of most practice management software programs and includes buttons that provide access to specific areas. Clicking on a specific button will allow you to work in that area of the program. Alternatively, there is an icon bar along the top left to quickly access the areas of the software, or the user may choose to navigate the software by using the pull-down menus below the software title bar.

- *Patient Registration:* allows you to input information about each patient in the practice, including demographic, HIPAA, and medical insurance information. From the Main Menu screen, click on the Patient Registration button to search for a patient, or to add a new patient, using the command buttons along the bottom of the patient selection dialog box.

- *Appointment Scheduling:* allows you to make appointments and also cancel, reschedule, and search for appointments. MOSS allows for block scheduling, as well as several print features including appointment cards and daily schedules.

- *Procedure Posting:* allows you to apply patient fees for services. When procedures are input into the procedure posting system, the software assigns the fee to be charged according to the fee schedule for the patient's insurance.

- *Insurance Billing:* allows you to prepare claims to be sent to insurance companies for the medical office to receive payment for services provided. You can generate and print a paper claim or simulate sending the claim electronically.

- *Claims Tracking:* simulates receiving an electronic explanation of benefits (EOB) or remittance advice (RA) from an insurance carrier.

- *Posting Payments:* allows you to input payments received by the practice from patients or insurance companies, as well as enter adjustments to the account.

- *Patient Billing:* allows you to generate a bill to be sent directly to the patient to collect any outstanding balances.

- *File Maintenance:* this is a utility area of the program that contains common information used by various systems within the software. In this area, you can create and restore Backup Files, change your password, turn Feedback Mode and Balloon Help on and off, and more.

CREATING BACKUP FILES

Backing up your MOSS database is just like saving a document or other file on your computer. Creating a backup file allows you to save all of the work you've completed up until that point. You may create a backup file of the work you've completed in the program at any time.

Backup files are very useful; for example, if you realize you have made a mistake and cannot correct it, you could restore a previous backup file and start the exercise over again. (Directions for restoring backup files are in the next section.)

For best results, we recommend creating a backup file after each Job requiring MOSS. Follow these steps to create a backup file:

1. Click on File Maintenance, and then click the button next to 2. Backup Database.
2. Click Yes at the prompt.
3. Now, select a location to save your backup file. We recommend that you save the database on a flash drive (in most computers, this is your E:/ or F:/ computer drive). When saving your file, you may also choose to rename the file. You may rename the file to anything you choose; however, you must keep the file extension (.mde) in the file name.

4. Click Save when you are finished. You will receive a prompt telling you that your file was completed successfully. Click OK.

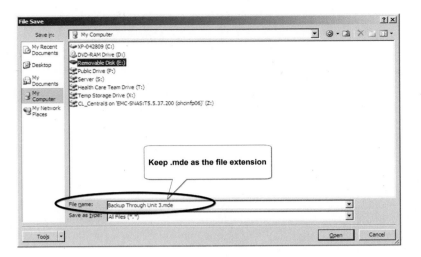

Restoring Backup Files

The restore function allows you to return to a previous point in the program. For instance, if you realize you have made a mistake and cannot correct it, you could restore a previous backup file and start the exercise over again. You may restore a backup file of previous work you've saved in the program at any time. Please note that restoring a backup file is permanent; all entries you have entered after creating that backup file will no longer appear in the program.

Follow these steps to restore a backup file:

1. Click on File Maintenance, and then click the button next to 3. Restore Database. Note that restoring a backup file is an irreversible process.
2. Click Yes at the prompt.
3. Click Restore MOSS from Database at the next prompt.
4. Click Yes at the following prompt. (Remember that restoring a backup file is an irreversible process.)
5. Find the backup file that you've created, click once to highlight it, and then click OK.
6. Click Yes at the following prompt.
7. Click the button Return to MOSS.
8. You have successfully restored your backup database. You will need to log in to the new database to start working.

Monday

March 4

9 00	Margaret Chandler	NP Chest pain	555-3423	FlexiHealth
9 15				
9 30				
9 45				
10 00	Pamela Cameron	NP Painful urination, tired	555-3510	UHC
10 15				
10 30				
10 45				
11 00	Walter Adams	BP Check	555-6836	Medicare
11 15				
11 30				
11 45				
12 00				
12 15		LUNCH		
12 30				
12 45				
1 00	Maureen Michaels	NP Asthmatic bronchitis	555-3258	Self-pay
1 15				
1 30				
1 45	Eric Garcia	Blood sugar test	555-4090	FlexiHealth
2 00	Raymond O'Neill	Return visit acute bronchitis	555-8453	Medicaid
2 15	Michele McLoud	Ear pain	555-2150	Self-pay
2 30				
2 45				
3 00				
3 15				
3 30		HOSPITAL		
3 45		ROUNDS		
4 00				
4 15				
4 30				
4 45				
5 00	**STAFF DINNER**			

Tuesday

March 5

Time	Name	Reason	Phone	Insurance
9 00				
9 15	STAFF BREAKFAST MEETING			
9 30				
9 45				
10 00	Susan Deng	Sore throat	555–8047	Prudential
10 15	Anna Miller	NP non-productive cough	555–4790	Medicare
10 30				
10 45				
11 00				
11 15	Bryan Lake	Blood pressure check	555-0327	Pacific
11 30	Nancy Talbot	Exam gastroententis	555–7317	FlexiHealth
11 45				
12 00				
12 15	**LUNCH**			
12 30				
12 45				
1 00	Tracey Mascello	Flu shot	555–1009	Self-pay
1 15	Elena Blanco	NP GYN exam	555–2659	FlexiHealth
1 30				
1 45				
2 00				
2 15	Thomas Smith	Recheck BP/allergy shot	555–6498	FlexiHealth
2 30	Aimee Bradley	Red, watery eyes	457–1446	ConsumerOne
2 45				
3 00				
3 15				
3 30				
3 45				
4 00				
4 15	Lecture at Douglasville			
4 30	Community College			
4 45				
5 00				

Wednesday
March 6

9 00				
9 15				
9 30	Leonard Mathers	Exam indigestion	555–4814	FlexiHealth
9 45				
10 00				
10 15				
10 30	Jessie Montgomery	Exam asthmatic bronchitis	555–1341	Medicare
10 45				
11 00				
11 15	Nancy Herbert	Recheck UTI	427–1133	Medicare Statewide
11 30		**Emergency slots**		
11 45				
12 00				
12 15		**Lunch Seminar**		
12 30		**at Hospital**		
12 45				
1 00				
1 15				
1 30				
1 45				
2 00				
2 15				
2 30				
2 45				
3 00				
3 15				
3 30				
3 45				
4 00				
4 15				
4 30				
4 45				
5 00				

	Thursday			
	March 7			
9 00				
9 15				
9 30				
9 45				
10 00				
10 15				
10 30				
10 45				
11 00	Xao Chang	CP	528–0112	Medicare Statewide
11 15				
11 30				
11 45				
12 00				
12 15		**LUNCH**		
12 30				
12 45				
1 00				
1 15	Deanna Hartsfeld	Exam Headache	457–6631	Medicare Statewide
1 30	**Emergency slots**			
1 45				
2 00				
2 15				
2 30	Dolores Perez	Blood pressure check	555–9772	Medicare
2 45				
3 00				
3 15				
3 30				
3 45				
4 00				
4 15				
4 30				
4 45				
5 00	Hospital Staff Meeting			

	Friday
	March 8

9 00				
9 15	Megan Caldwell	Exam UTI	458–2839	FlexiHealth
9 30				
9 45				
10 00		**Emergency slots**		
10 15				
10 30				
10 45				
11 00				
11 15				
11 30				
11 45				
12 00				
12 15		**LUNCH**		
12 30				
12 45				
1 00				
1 15				
1 30				
1 45				
2 00	Walter Adams	Exam BP check	555–6836	Medicare
2 15				
2 30				
2 45				
3 00				
3 15				
3 30				
3 45				
4 00				
4 15		HOSPITAL		
4 30		ROUNDS		
4 45				
5 00				

Monday
March 11

9 00	
9 15	
9 30	
9 45	
10 00	
10 15	
10 30	
10 45	
11 00	
11 15	
11 30	
11 45	
12 00	
12 15	LUNCH
12 30	
12 45	
1 00	
1 15	
1 30	
1 45	
2 00	
2 15	
2 30	
2 45	
3 00	
3 15	
3 30	
3 45	
4 00	
4 15	
4 30	
4 45	
5 00	

Patient List
Tuesday
March 5

Hour	Patient	Procedure	Nature of Illness	Time
9 00				
9 15				
9 30				
9 45				
10 00				
10 15				
10 30				
10 45				
11 00				
11 15				
11 30				
11 45				
12 00				
12 15				
12 30				
12 45				
1 00				
1 15				
1 30				
1 45				
2 00				
2 15				
2 30				
2 45				
3 00				
3 15				
3 30				
3 45				
4 00				
4 15				
4 30				
4 45				
5 00				

Patient List
Wednesday
March 6

Hour	Patient	Procedure	Nature of Illness	Time
9 00				
9 15				
9 30				
9 45				
10 00				
10 15				
10 30				
10 45				
11 00				
11 15				
11 30				
11 45				
12 00				
12 15				
12 30				
12 45				
1 00				
1 15				
1 30				
1 45				
2 00				
2 15				
2 30				
2 45				
3 00				
3 15				
3 30				
3 45				
4 00				
4 15				
4 30				
4 45				
5 00				

Patient List
Thursday
March 7

Hour	Patient	Procedure	Nature of Illness	Time
9 00				
9 15				
9 30				
9 45				
10 00				
10 15				
10 30				
10 45				
11 00				
11 15				
11 30				
11 45				
12 00				
12 15				
12 30				
12 45				
1 00				
1 15				
1 30				
1 45				
2 00				
2 15				
2 30				
2 45				
3 00				
3 15				
3 30				
3 45				
4 00				
4 15				
4 30				
4 45				
5 00				

Patient List
Friday
March 8

Hour	Patient	Procedure	Nature of Illness	Time
9 00				
9 15				
9 30				
9 45				
10 00				
10 15				
10 30				
10 45				
11 00				
11 15				
11 30				
11 45				
12 00				
12 15				
12 30				
12 45				
1 00				
1 15				
1 30				
1 45				
2 00				
2 15				
2 30				
2 45				
3 00				
3 15				
3 30				
3 45				
4 00				
4 15				
4 30				
4 45				
5 00				

Patient List
Monday
March 11

Hour	Patient	Procedure	Nature of Illness	Time
9 00				
9 15				
9 30				
9 45				
10 00				
10 15				
10 30				
10 45				
11 00				
11 15				
11 30				
11 45				
12 00				
12 15				
12 30				
12 45				
1 00				
1 15				
1 30				
1 45				
2 00				
2 15				
2 30				
2 45				
3 00				
3 15				
3 30				
3 45				
4 00				
4 15				
4 30				
4 45				
5 00				

1500

HEALTH INSURANCE CLAIM FORM

APPROVED BY NATIONAL UNIFORM CLAIM COMMITTEE 08/05

| | | PICA | | | | | | | | PICA | | | |

1. MEDICARE (Medicare #) **MEDICAID** (Medicaid #) **TRICARE CHAMPUS** (Sponsor's SSN) **CHAMPVA** (Member ID#) **GROUP HEALTH PLAN** (SSN or ID) **FECA BLK LUNG** (SSN) **OTHER** (ID)

1a. INSURED'S I.D. NUMBER (For Program in Item 1)

2. PATIENT'S NAME (Last Name, First Name, Middle Initial)

3. PATIENT'S BIRTH DATE MM DD YY   **SEX** M   F

4. INSURED'S NAME (Last Name, First Name, Middle Initial)

5. PATIENT'S ADDRESS (No., Street)

6. PATIENT RELATIONSHIP TO INSURED Self   Spouse   Child   Other

7. INSURED'S ADDRESS (No., Street)

CITY   STATE

8. PATIENT STATUS Single   Married   Other

Employed   Full-Time Student   Part-Time Student

CITY   STATE

ZIP CODE   **TELEPHONE** (Include Area Code) ( )

ZIP CODE   **TELEPHONE** (Include Area Code) ( )

9. OTHER INSURED'S NAME (Last Name, First Name, Middle Initial)

10. IS PATIENT'S CONDITION RELATED TO:

11. INSURED'S POLICY GROUP OR FECA NUMBER

a. OTHER INSURED'S POLICY OR GROUP NUMBER

a. EMPLOYMENT? (Current or Previous) YES   NO

a. INSURED'S DATE OF BIRTH MM DD YY   **SEX** M   F

b. OTHER INSURED'S DATE OF BIRTH MM DD YY   **SEX** M   F

b. AUTO ACCIDENT? YES   NO   PLACE (State)

b. EMPLOYER'S NAME OR SCHOOL NAME

c. EMPLOYER'S NAME OR SCHOOL NAME

c. OTHER ACCIDENT? YES   NO

c. INSURANCE PLAN NAME OR PROGRAM NAME

d. INSURANCE PLAN NAME OR PROGRAM NAME

10d. RESERVED FOR LOCAL USE

d. IS THERE ANOTHER HEALTH BENEFIT PLAN? YES   NO   *If yes, return to and complete item 9 a-d.*

READ BACK OF FORM BEFORE COMPLETING & SIGNING THIS FORM.
12. PATIENT'S OR AUTHORIZED PERSON'S SIGNATURE I authorize the release of any medical or other information necessary to process this claim. I also request payment of government benefits either to myself or to the party who accepts assignment below.

SIGNED _____ DATE _____

13. INSURED'S OR AUTHORIZED PERSON'S SIGNATURE I authorize payment of medical benefits to the undersigned physician or supplier for services described below.

SIGNED _____

14. DATE OF CURRENT: MM DD YY   ILLNESS (First symptom) OR INJURY (Accident) OR PREGNANCY(LMP)

15. IF PATIENT HAS HAD SAME OR SIMILAR ILLNESS. GIVE FIRST DATE MM DD YY

16. DATES PATIENT UNABLE TO WORK IN CURRENT OCCUPATION FROM MM DD YY   TO MM DD YY

17. NAME OF REFERRING PROVIDER OR OTHER SOURCE   17a.   17b. NPI

18. HOSPITALIZATION DATES RELATED TO CURRENT SERVICES FROM MM DD YY   TO MM DD YY

19. RESERVED FOR LOCAL USE

20. OUTSIDE LAB? YES   NO $ CHARGES

21. DIAGNOSIS OR NATURE OF ILLNESS OR INJURY (Relate Items 1, 2, 3 or 4 to Item 24E by Line)
1. |___.___   3. |___.___
2. |___.___   4. |___.___

22. MEDICAID RESUBMISSION CODE   ORIGINAL REF. NO.

23. PRIOR AUTHORIZATION NUMBER

24. A. DATE(S) OF SERVICE						B. PLACE OF SERVICE	C. EMG	D. PROCEDURES, SERVICES, OR SUPPLIES (Explain Unusual Circumstances)		E. DIAGNOSIS POINTER	F. $ CHARGES	G. DAYS OR UNITS	H. EPSDT Family Plan	I. ID. QUAL.	J. RENDERING PROVIDER ID. #
From MM	DD	YY	To MM	DD	YY			CPT/HCPCS	MODIFIER						
1														NPI	
2														NPI	
3														NPI	
4														NPI	
5														NPI	
6														NPI	

25. FEDERAL TAX I.D. NUMBER   SSN EIN

26. PATIENT'S ACCOUNT NO.

27. ACCEPT ASSIGNMENT? (For govt. claims, see back) YES   NO

28. TOTAL CHARGE $

29. AMOUNT PAID $

30. BALANCE DUE $

31. SIGNATURE OF PHYSICIAN OR SUPPLIER INCLUDING DEGREES OR CREDENTIALS (I certify that the statements on the reverse apply to this bill and are made a part thereof.)

SIGNED _____ DATE _____

32. SERVICE FACILITY LOCATION INFORMATION

a. NPI   b.

33. BILLING PROVIDER INFO & PH # (123) 456-7890
DOUGLASVILLE MEDICINE ASSOCIATES
5076 BRAND BLVD, STE 401
DOUGLASVILLE, NY 01234
a. 9995010111   b.

NUCC Instruction Manual available at: www.nucc.org

APPROVED OMB-0938-0999 FORM CMS-1500 (08/05)

(vertical right margin: CARRIER — PATIENT AND INSURED INFORMATION — PHYSICIAN OR SUPPLIER INFORMATION)

1500

HEALTH INSURANCE CLAIM FORM

APPROVED BY NATIONAL UNIFORM CLAIM COMMITTEE 08/05

PICA		PICA

1. MEDICARE	MEDICAID	TRICARE CHAMPUS	CHAMPVA	GROUP HEALTH PLAN	FECA BLK LUNG	OTHER	1a. INSURED'S I.D. NUMBER (For Program in Item 1)
(Medicare #)	(Medicaid #)	(Sponsor's SSN)	(Member ID#)	(SSN or ID)	(SSN)	(ID)	

2. PATIENT'S NAME (Last Name, First Name, Middle Initial)

3. PATIENT'S BIRTH DATE MM DD YY   SEX M F

4. INSURED'S NAME (Last Name, First Name, Middle Initial)

5. PATIENT'S ADDRESS (No., Street)

6. PATIENT RELATIONSHIP TO INSURED   Self Spouse Child Other

7. INSURED'S ADDRESS (No., Street)

CITY   STATE

8. PATIENT STATUS   Single Married Other

CITY   STATE

ZIP CODE   TELEPHONE (Include Area Code) ( )

Employed Full-Time Student Part-Time Student

ZIP CODE   TELEPHONE (Include Area Code) ( )

9. OTHER INSURED'S NAME (Last Name, First Name, Middle Initial)

10. IS PATIENT'S CONDITION RELATED TO:

11. INSURED'S POLICY GROUP OR FECA NUMBER

a. OTHER INSURED'S POLICY OR GROUP NUMBER

a. EMPLOYMENT? (Current or Previous) YES NO

a. INSURED'S DATE OF BIRTH MM DD YY   SEX M F

b. OTHER INSURED'S DATE OF BIRTH MM DD YY   SEX M F

b. AUTO ACCIDENT? YES NO   PLACE (State)

b. EMPLOYER'S NAME OR SCHOOL NAME

c. EMPLOYER'S NAME OR SCHOOL NAME

c. OTHER ACCIDENT? YES NO

c. INSURANCE PLAN NAME OR PROGRAM NAME

d. INSURANCE PLAN NAME OR PROGRAM NAME

10d. RESERVED FOR LOCAL USE

d. IS THERE ANOTHER HEALTH BENEFIT PLAN? YES NO   If yes, return to and complete item 9 a-d.

READ BACK OF FORM BEFORE COMPLETING & SIGNING THIS FORM.
12. PATIENT'S OR AUTHORIZED PERSON'S SIGNATURE I authorize the release of any medical or other information necessary to process this claim. I also request payment of government benefits either to myself or to the party who accepts assignment below.

SIGNED _____ DATE _____

13. INSURED'S OR AUTHORIZED PERSON'S SIGNATURE I authorize payment of medical benefits to the undersigned physician or supplier for services described below.

SIGNED _____

14. DATE OF CURRENT: MM DD YY ILLNESS (First symptom) OR INJURY (Accident) OR PREGNANCY(LMP)

15. IF PATIENT HAS HAD SAME OR SIMILAR ILLNESS. GIVE FIRST DATE MM DD YY

16. DATES PATIENT UNABLE TO WORK IN CURRENT OCCUPATION MM DD YY FROM   TO MM DD YY

17. NAME OF REFERRING PROVIDER OR OTHER SOURCE

17a.
17b. NPI

18. HOSPITALIZATION DATES RELATED TO CURRENT SERVICES MM DD YY FROM   TO MM DD YY

19. RESERVED FOR LOCAL USE

20. OUTSIDE LAB? YES NO $ CHARGES

21. DIAGNOSIS OR NATURE OF ILLNESS OR INJURY (Relate Items 1, 2, 3 or 4 to Item 24E by Line)

1. _____   3. _____
2. _____   4. _____

22. MEDICAID RESUBMISSION CODE   ORIGINAL REF. NO.

23. PRIOR AUTHORIZATION NUMBER

24. A. DATE(S) OF SERVICE From MM DD YY To MM DD YY	B. PLACE OF SERVICE	C. EMG	D. PROCEDURES, SERVICES, OR SUPPLIES (Explain Unusual Circumstances) CPT/HCPCS MODIFIER	E. DIAGNOSIS POINTER	F. $ CHARGES	G. DAYS OR UNITS	H. EPSDT Family Plan	I. ID. QUAL.	J. RENDERING PROVIDER ID. #
1								NPI	
2								NPI	
3								NPI	
4								NPI	
5								NPI	
6								NPI	

25. FEDERAL TAX I.D. NUMBER   SSN EIN

26. PATIENT'S ACCOUNT NO.

27. ACCEPT ASSIGNMENT? (For govt. claims, see back) YES NO

28. TOTAL CHARGE $

29. AMOUNT PAID $

30. BALANCE DUE $

31. SIGNATURE OF PHYSICIAN OR SUPPLIER INCLUDING DEGREES OR CREDENTIALS (I certify that the statements on the reverse apply to this bill and are made a part thereof.)

SIGNED _____ DATE _____

32. SERVICE FACILITY LOCATION INFORMATION

a. NPI   b.

33. BILLING PROVIDER INFO & PH # (123) 456-7890
DOUGLASVILLE MEDICINE ASSOCIATES
5076 BRAND BLVD, STE 401
DOUGLASVILLE, NY 01234
a. 9995010111   b.

NUCC Instruction Manual available at: www.nucc.org

APPROVED OMB-0938-0999 FORM CMS-1500 (08/05)

CARRIER

PATIENT AND INSURED INFORMATION

PHYSICIAN OR SUPPLIER INFORMATION

1500

HEALTH INSURANCE CLAIM FORM

APPROVED BY NATIONAL UNIFORM CLAIM COMMITTEE 08/05

PICA | | PICA

1. MEDICARE ☐ (Medicare #) MEDICAID ☐ (Medicaid #) TRICARE CHAMPUS ☐ (Sponsor's SSN) CHAMPVA ☐ (Member ID#) GROUP HEALTH PLAN ☐ (SSN or ID) FECA BLK LUNG ☐ (SSN) OTHER ☐ (ID) | 1a. INSURED'S I.D. NUMBER (For Program in Item 1)

2. PATIENT'S NAME (Last Name, First Name, Middle Initial)

3. PATIENT'S BIRTH DATE MM DD YY   SEX M ☐ F ☐

4. INSURED'S NAME (Last Name, First Name, Middle Initial)

5. PATIENT'S ADDRESS (No., Street)

6. PATIENT RELATIONSHIP TO INSURED Self ☐ Spouse ☐ Child ☐ Other ☐

7. INSURED'S ADDRESS (No., Street)

CITY   STATE

8. PATIENT STATUS Single ☐ Married ☐ Other ☐

CITY   STATE

ZIP CODE   TELEPHONE (Include Area Code) ( )

Employed ☐ Full-Time Student ☐ Part-Time Student ☐

ZIP CODE   TELEPHONE (Include Area Code) ( )

9. OTHER INSURED'S NAME (Last Name, First Name, Middle Initial)

10. IS PATIENT'S CONDITION RELATED TO:

11. INSURED'S POLICY GROUP OR FECA NUMBER

a. OTHER INSURED'S POLICY OR GROUP NUMBER

a. EMPLOYMENT? (Current or Previous) YES ☐ NO ☐

a. INSURED'S DATE OF BIRTH MM DD YY   SEX M ☐ F ☐

b. OTHER INSURED'S DATE OF BIRTH MM DD YY   SEX M ☐ F ☐

b. AUTO ACCIDENT?   PLACE (State) YES ☐ NO ☐

b. EMPLOYER'S NAME OR SCHOOL NAME

c. EMPLOYER'S NAME OR SCHOOL NAME

c. OTHER ACCIDENT? YES ☐ NO ☐

c. INSURANCE PLAN NAME OR PROGRAM NAME

d. INSURANCE PLAN NAME OR PROGRAM NAME

10d. RESERVED FOR LOCAL USE

d. IS THERE ANOTHER HEALTH BENEFIT PLAN? YES ☐ NO ☐ If yes, return to and complete item 9 a-d.

READ BACK OF FORM BEFORE COMPLETING & SIGNING THIS FORM.
12. PATIENT'S OR AUTHORIZED PERSON'S SIGNATURE I authorize the release of any medical or other information necessary to process this claim. I also request payment of government benefits either to myself or to the party who accepts assignment below.

SIGNED _____   DATE _____

13. INSURED'S OR AUTHORIZED PERSON'S SIGNATURE I authorize payment of medical benefits to the undersigned physician or supplier for services described below.

SIGNED _____

14. DATE OF CURRENT: MM DD YY ◄ ILLNESS (First symptom) OR INJURY (Accident) OR PREGNANCY(LMP)

15. IF PATIENT HAS HAD SAME OR SIMILAR ILLNESS. GIVE FIRST DATE MM DD YY

16. DATES PATIENT UNABLE TO WORK IN CURRENT OCCUPATION FROM MM DD YY   TO MM DD YY

17. NAME OF REFERRING PROVIDER OR OTHER SOURCE

17a.
17b. NPI

18. HOSPITALIZATION DATES RELATED TO CURRENT SERVICES FROM MM DD YY   TO MM DD YY

19. RESERVED FOR LOCAL USE

20. OUTSIDE LAB? YES ☐ NO ☐ $ CHARGES

21. DIAGNOSIS OR NATURE OF ILLNESS OR INJURY (Relate Items 1, 2, 3 or 4 to Item 24E by Line)

1. |___.___
2. |___.___
3. |___.___
4. |___.___

22. MEDICAID RESUBMISSION CODE   ORIGINAL REF. NO.

23. PRIOR AUTHORIZATION NUMBER

24. A. DATE(S) OF SERVICE						B. PLACE OF SERVICE	C. EMG	D. PROCEDURES, SERVICES, OR SUPPLIES (Explain Unusual Circumstances)		E. DIAGNOSIS POINTER	F. $ CHARGES	G. DAYS OR UNITS	H. EPSDT Family Plan	I. ID. QUAL.	J. RENDERING PROVIDER ID. #
From			To					CPT/HCPCS	MODIFIER						
MM	DD	YY	MM	DD	YY										
1														NPI	
2														NPI	
3														NPI	
4														NPI	
5														NPI	
6														NPI	

25. FEDERAL TAX I.D. NUMBER   SSN ☐ EIN ☐

26. PATIENT'S ACCOUNT NO.

27. ACCEPT ASSIGNMENT? (For govt. claims, see back) YES ☐ NO ☐

28. TOTAL CHARGE $

29. AMOUNT PAID $

30. BALANCE DUE $

31. SIGNATURE OF PHYSICIAN OR SUPPLIER INCLUDING DEGREES OR CREDENTIALS (I certify that the statements on the reverse apply to this bill and are made a part thereof.)

SIGNED _____ DATE _____

32. SERVICE FACILITY LOCATION INFORMATION

a. NPI   b.

33. BILLING PROVIDER INFO & PH # (123) 456-7890
DOUGLASVILLE MEDICINE ASSOCIATES
5076 BRAND BLVD, STE 401
DOUGLASVILLE, NY 01234

a. 9995010111   b.

NUCC Instruction Manual available at: www.nucc.org

APPROVED OMB-0938-0999 FORM CMS-1500 (08/05)

Right margin (vertical): CARRIER → · PATIENT AND INSURED INFORMATION · PHYSICIAN OR SUPPLIER INFORMATION

1500

HEALTH INSURANCE CLAIM FORM

APPROVED BY NATIONAL UNIFORM CLAIM COMMITTEE 08/05

| | PICA | | | | | | | | | PICA | |

| 1. MEDICARE | MEDICAID | TRICARE CHAMPUS | CHAMPVA | GROUP HEALTH PLAN | FECA BLK LUNG | OTHER | 1a. INSURED'S I.D. NUMBER | (For Program in Item 1) |
| (Medicare #) | (Medicaid #) | (Sponsor's SSN) | (Member ID#) | (SSN or ID) | (SSN) | (ID) | | |

2. PATIENT'S NAME (Last Name, First Name, Middle Initial)

3. PATIENT'S BIRTH DATE MM DD YY   SEX   M   F

4. INSURED'S NAME (Last Name, First Name, Middle Initial)

5. PATIENT'S ADDRESS (No., Street)

6. PATIENT RELATIONSHIP TO INSURED   Self   Spouse   Child   Other

7. INSURED'S ADDRESS (No., Street)

CITY   STATE

8. PATIENT STATUS   Single   Married   Other

CITY   STATE

ZIP CODE   TELEPHONE (Include Area Code) ( )

Employed   Full-Time Student   Part-Time Student

ZIP CODE   TELEPHONE (Include Area Code) ( )

9. OTHER INSURED'S NAME (Last Name, First Name, Middle Initial)

10. IS PATIENT'S CONDITION RELATED TO:

11. INSURED'S POLICY GROUP OR FECA NUMBER

a. OTHER INSURED'S POLICY OR GROUP NUMBER

a. EMPLOYMENT? (Current or Previous)   YES   NO

a. INSURED'S DATE OF BIRTH MM DD YY   SEX   M   F

b. OTHER INSURED'S DATE OF BIRTH MM DD YY   SEX   M   F

b. AUTO ACCIDENT?   PLACE (State)   YES   NO

b. EMPLOYER'S NAME OR SCHOOL NAME

c. EMPLOYER'S NAME OR SCHOOL NAME

c. OTHER ACCIDENT?   YES   NO

c. INSURANCE PLAN NAME OR PROGRAM NAME

d. INSURANCE PLAN NAME OR PROGRAM NAME

10d. RESERVED FOR LOCAL USE

d. IS THERE ANOTHER HEALTH BENEFIT PLAN?   YES   NO   If yes, return to and complete Item 9 a-d.

READ BACK OF FORM BEFORE COMPLETING & SIGNING THIS FORM.

12. PATIENT'S OR AUTHORIZED PERSON'S SIGNATURE I authorize the release of any medical or other information necessary to process this claim. I also request payment of government benefits either to myself or to the party who accepts assignment below.

SIGNED _____   DATE _____

13. INSURED'S OR AUTHORIZED PERSON'S SIGNATURE I authorize payment of medical benefits to the undersigned physician or supplier for services described below.

SIGNED _____

14. DATE OF CURRENT: MM DD YY   ILLNESS (First symptom) OR INJURY (Accident) OR PREGNANCY(LMP)

15. IF PATIENT HAS HAD SAME OR SIMILAR ILLNESS. GIVE FIRST DATE MM DD YY

16. DATES PATIENT UNABLE TO WORK IN CURRENT OCCUPATION FROM MM DD YY   TO MM DD YY

17. NAME OF REFERRING PROVIDER OR OTHER SOURCE

17a.

17b. NPI

18. HOSPITALIZATION DATES RELATED TO CURRENT SERVICES FROM MM DD YY   TO MM DD YY

19. RESERVED FOR LOCAL USE

20. OUTSIDE LAB?   YES   NO $ CHARGES

21. DIAGNOSIS OR NATURE OF ILLNESS OR INJURY (Relate Items 1, 2, 3 or 4 to Item 24E by Line)

1. ____ . ____   3. ____ . ____

2. ____ . ____   4. ____ . ____

22. MEDICAID RESUBMISSION CODE   ORIGINAL REF. NO.

23. PRIOR AUTHORIZATION NUMBER

24. A. DATE(S) OF SERVICE			B. PLACE OF	C.	D. PROCEDURES, SERVICES, OR SUPPLIES		E. DIAGNOSIS	F.	G. DAYS OR	H. EPSDT Family	I.	J. RENDERING
From		To	SERVICE	EMG	(Explain Unusual Circumstances)		POINTER	$ CHARGES	UNITS	Plan	ID. QUAL.	PROVIDER ID. #
MM DD YY	MM DD YY				CPT/HCPCS	MODIFIER						
1											NPI	
2											NPI	
3											NPI	
4											NPI	
5											NPI	
6											NPI	

25. FEDERAL TAX I.D. NUMBER   SSN EIN

26. PATIENT'S ACCOUNT NO.

27. ACCEPT ASSIGNMENT? (For govt. claims, see back)   YES   NO

28. TOTAL CHARGE $

29. AMOUNT PAID $

30. BALANCE DUE $

31. SIGNATURE OF PHYSICIAN OR SUPPLIER INCLUDING DEGREES OR CREDENTIALS (I certify that the statements on the reverse apply to this bill and are made a part thereof.)

SIGNED _____   DATE _____

32. SERVICE FACILITY LOCATION INFORMATION

a. NPI   b.

33. BILLING PROVIDER INFO & PH # (123) 456-7890

DOUGLASVILLE MEDICINE ASSOCIATES
5076 BRAND BLVD, STE 401
DOUGLASVILLE, NY 01234

a. 9995010111   b.

NUCC Instruction Manual available at: www.nucc.org

APPROVED OMB-0938-0999 FORM CMS-1500 (08/05)

CARRIER

PATIENT AND INSURED INFORMATION

PHYSICIAN OR SUPPLIER INFORMATION

1500

HEALTH INSURANCE CLAIM FORM

APPROVED BY NATIONAL UNIFORM CLAIM COMMITTEE 08/05

☐☐ PICA

PICA ☐☐

1. MEDICARE	MEDICAID	TRICARE CHAMPUS	CHAMPVA	GROUP HEALTH PLAN	FECA BLK LUNG	OTHER	1a. INSURED'S I.D. NUMBER (For Program in Item 1)
☐ (Medicare #)	☐ (Medicaid #)	☐ (Sponsor's SSN)	☐ (Member ID#)	☐ (SSN or ID)	☐ (SSN)	☐ (ID)	

2. PATIENT'S NAME (Last Name, First Name, Middle Initial)

3. PATIENT'S BIRTH DATE MM DD YY | SEX M ☐ F ☐

4. INSURED'S NAME (Last Name, First Name, Middle Initial)

5. PATIENT'S ADDRESS (No., Street)

6. PATIENT RELATIONSHIP TO INSURED
Self ☐ Spouse ☐ Child ☐ Other ☐

7. INSURED'S ADDRESS (No., Street)

CITY | STATE

8. PATIENT STATUS
Single ☐ Married ☐ Other ☐
Employed ☐ Full-Time Student ☐ Part-Time Student ☐

CITY | STATE

ZIP CODE | TELEPHONE (Include Area Code) ( )

ZIP CODE | TELEPHONE (Include Area Code) ( )

9. OTHER INSURED'S NAME (Last Name, First Name, Middle Initial)

10. IS PATIENT'S CONDITION RELATED TO:

11. INSURED'S POLICY GROUP OR FECA NUMBER

a. OTHER INSURED'S POLICY OR GROUP NUMBER

a. EMPLOYMENT? (Current or Previous)
☐ YES ☐ NO

a. INSURED'S DATE OF BIRTH MM DD YY | SEX M ☐ F ☐

b. OTHER INSURED'S DATE OF BIRTH MM DD YY | SEX M ☐ F ☐

b. AUTO ACCIDENT? PLACE (State)
☐ YES ☐ NO

b. EMPLOYER'S NAME OR SCHOOL NAME

c. EMPLOYER'S NAME OR SCHOOL NAME

c. OTHER ACCIDENT?
☐ YES ☐ NO

c. INSURANCE PLAN NAME OR PROGRAM NAME

d. INSURANCE PLAN NAME OR PROGRAM NAME

10d. RESERVED FOR LOCAL USE

d. IS THERE ANOTHER HEALTH BENEFIT PLAN?
☐ YES ☐ NO If yes, return to and complete item 9 a-d.

READ BACK OF FORM BEFORE COMPLETING & SIGNING THIS FORM.
12. PATIENT'S OR AUTHORIZED PERSON'S SIGNATURE I authorize the release of any medical or other information necessary to process this claim. I also request payment of government benefits either to myself or to the party who accepts assignment below.

SIGNED _____ DATE _____

13. INSURED'S OR AUTHORIZED PERSON'S SIGNATURE I authorize payment of medical benefits to the undersigned physician or supplier for services described below.

SIGNED _____

14. DATE OF CURRENT: MM DD YY ◄ ILLNESS (First symptom) OR INJURY (Accident) OR PREGNANCY(LMP)

15. IF PATIENT HAS HAD SAME OR SIMILAR ILLNESS. GIVE FIRST DATE MM DD YY

16. DATES PATIENT UNABLE TO WORK IN CURRENT OCCUPATION FROM MM DD YY TO MM DD YY

17. NAME OF REFERRING PROVIDER OR OTHER SOURCE | 17a. | 17b. NPI

18. HOSPITALIZATION DATES RELATED TO CURRENT SERVICES FROM MM DD YY TO MM DD YY

19. RESERVED FOR LOCAL USE

20. OUTSIDE LAB? ☐ YES ☐ NO | $ CHARGES

21. DIAGNOSIS OR NATURE OF ILLNESS OR INJURY (Relate Items 1, 2, 3 or 4 to Item 24E by Line)
1. |___.___| 3. |___.___|
2. |___.___| 4. |___.___|

22. MEDICAID RESUBMISSION CODE | ORIGINAL REF. NO.

23. PRIOR AUTHORIZATION NUMBER

24. A. DATE(S) OF SERVICE						B. PLACE OF SERVICE	C. EMG	D. PROCEDURES, SERVICES, OR SUPPLIES (Explain Unusual Circumstances) CPT/HCPCS	MODIFIER	E. DIAGNOSIS POINTER	F. $ CHARGES	G. DAYS OR UNITS	H. EPSDT Family Plan	I. ID. QUAL.	J. RENDERING PROVIDER ID. #
From MM	DD	YY	To MM	DD	YY										
1														NPI	
2														NPI	
3														NPI	
4														NPI	
5														NPI	
6														NPI	

25. FEDERAL TAX I.D. NUMBER ☐ SSN ☐ EIN

26. PATIENT'S ACCOUNT NO.

27. ACCEPT ASSIGNMENT? (For govt. claims, see back) ☐ YES ☐ NO

28. TOTAL CHARGE $

29. AMOUNT PAID $

30. BALANCE DUE $

31. SIGNATURE OF PHYSICIAN OR SUPPLIER INCLUDING DEGREES OR CREDENTIALS (I certify that the statements on the reverse apply to this bill and are made a part thereof.)

SIGNED _____ DATE _____

32. SERVICE FACILITY LOCATION INFORMATION
a. NPI   b.

33. BILLING PROVIDER INFO & PH # (123) 456-7890
DOUGLASVILLE MEDICINE ASSOCIATES
5076 BRAND BLVD, STE 401
DOUGLASVILLE, NY 01234
a. 9995010111   b.

NUCC Instruction Manual available at: www.nucc.org

APPROVED OMB-0938-0999 FORM CMS-1500 (08/05)

1500

HEALTH INSURANCE CLAIM FORM

APPROVED BY NATIONAL UNIFORM CLAIM COMMITTEE 08/05

PICA

CARRIER

1. MEDICARE MEDICAID TRICARE CHAMPVA GROUP FECA OTHER	1a. INSURED'S I.D. NUMBER (For Program in Item 1)

1. MEDICARE (Medicare #) MEDICAID (Medicaid #) TRICARE CHAMPUS (Sponsor's SSN) CHAMPVA (Member ID#) GROUP HEALTH PLAN (SSN or ID) FECA BLK LUNG (SSN) OTHER (ID)

1a. INSURED'S I.D. NUMBER (For Program in Item 1)

2. PATIENT'S NAME (Last Name, First Name, Middle Initial)

3. PATIENT'S BIRTH DATE MM DD YY   SEX M F

4. INSURED'S NAME (Last Name, First Name, Middle Initial)

5. PATIENT'S ADDRESS (No., Street)

6. PATIENT RELATIONSHIP TO INSURED   Self Spouse Child Other

7. INSURED'S ADDRESS (No., Street)

CITY   STATE

8. PATIENT STATUS   Single Married Other

CITY   STATE

ZIP CODE   TELEPHONE (Include Area Code) (   )

Employed Full-Time Student Part-Time Student

ZIP CODE   TELEPHONE (Include Area Code) (   )

9. OTHER INSURED'S NAME (Last Name, First Name, Middle Initial)

10. IS PATIENT'S CONDITION RELATED TO:

11. INSURED'S POLICY GROUP OR FECA NUMBER

a. OTHER INSURED'S POLICY OR GROUP NUMBER

a. EMPLOYMENT? (Current or Previous) YES NO

a. INSURED'S DATE OF BIRTH MM DD YY   SEX M F

b. OTHER INSURED'S DATE OF BIRTH MM DD YY   SEX M F

b. AUTO ACCIDENT? YES NO   PLACE (State)

b. EMPLOYER'S NAME OR SCHOOL NAME

c. EMPLOYER'S NAME OR SCHOOL NAME

c. OTHER ACCIDENT? YES NO

c. INSURANCE PLAN NAME OR PROGRAM NAME

d. INSURANCE PLAN NAME OR PROGRAM NAME

10d. RESERVED FOR LOCAL USE

d. IS THERE ANOTHER HEALTH BENEFIT PLAN? YES NO   *If yes*, return to and complete item 9 a-d.

PATIENT AND INSURED INFORMATION

READ BACK OF FORM BEFORE COMPLETING & SIGNING THIS FORM.

12. PATIENT'S OR AUTHORIZED PERSON'S SIGNATURE I authorize the release of any medical or other information necessary to process this claim. I also request payment of government benefits either to myself or to the party who accepts assignment below.

SIGNED _____   DATE _____

13. INSURED'S OR AUTHORIZED PERSON'S SIGNATURE I authorize payment of medical benefits to the undersigned physician or supplier for services described below.

SIGNED _____

14. DATE OF CURRENT: MM DD YY   ILLNESS (First symptom) OR INJURY (Accident) OR PREGNANCY(LMP)

15. IF PATIENT HAS HAD SAME OR SIMILAR ILLNESS. GIVE FIRST DATE MM DD YY

16. DATES PATIENT UNABLE TO WORK IN CURRENT OCCUPATION MM DD YY   FROM   TO MM DD YY

17. NAME OF REFERRING PROVIDER OR OTHER SOURCE

17a.
17b. NPI

18. HOSPITALIZATION DATES RELATED TO CURRENT SERVICES MM DD YY   FROM   TO MM DD YY

19. RESERVED FOR LOCAL USE

20. OUTSIDE LAB? YES NO $ CHARGES

21. DIAGNOSIS OR NATURE OF ILLNESS OR INJURY (Relate Items 1, 2, 3 or 4 to Item 24E by Line)

1. ____ . ____   3. ____ . ____

2. ____ . ____   4. ____ . ____

22. MEDICAID RESUBMISSION CODE   ORIGINAL REF. NO.

23. PRIOR AUTHORIZATION NUMBER

24. A. DATE(S) OF SERVICE From MM DD YY To MM DD YY	B. PLACE OF SERVICE	C. EMG	D. PROCEDURES, SERVICES, OR SUPPLIES (Explain Unusual Circumstances) CPT/HCPCS MODIFIER	E. DIAGNOSIS POINTER	F. $ CHARGES	G. DAYS OR UNITS	H. EPSDT Family Plan	I. ID. QUAL.	J. RENDERING PROVIDER ID. #
1								NPI	
2								NPI	
3								NPI	
4								NPI	
5								NPI	
6								NPI	

PHYSICIAN OR SUPPLIER INFORMATION

25. FEDERAL TAX I.D. NUMBER   SSN EIN

26. PATIENT'S ACCOUNT NO.

27. ACCEPT ASSIGNMENT? (For govt. claims, see back) YES NO

28. TOTAL CHARGE $

29. AMOUNT PAID $

30. BALANCE DUE $

31. SIGNATURE OF PHYSICIAN OR SUPPLIER INCLUDING DEGREES OR CREDENTIALS (I certify that the statements on the reverse apply to this bill and are made a part thereof.)

SIGNED _____   DATE _____

32. SERVICE FACILITY LOCATION INFORMATION

a. NPI   b.

33. BILLING PROVIDER INFO & PH # (123) 456-7890

DOUGLASVILLE MEDICINE ASSOCIATES
5076 BRAND BLVD, STE 401
DOUGLASVILLE, NY 01234

a. 9995010111   b.

NUCC Instruction Manual available at: www.nucc.org

APPROVED OMB-0938-0999 FORM CMS-1500 (08/05)

1500

HEALTH INSURANCE CLAIM FORM

APPROVED BY NATIONAL UNIFORM CLAIM COMMITTEE 08/05

☐☐ PICA   PICA ☐☐

| 1. MEDICARE ☐ (Medicare #)   MEDICAID ☐ (Medicaid #)   TRICARE CHAMPUS ☐ (Sponsor's SSN)   CHAMPVA ☐ (Member ID#)   GROUP HEALTH PLAN ☐ (SSN or ID)   FECA BLK LUNG ☐ (SSN)   OTHER ☐ (ID) | 1a. INSURED'S I.D. NUMBER   (For Program in Item 1) |

| 2. PATIENT'S NAME (Last Name, First Name, Middle Initial) | 3. PATIENT'S BIRTH DATE MM DD YY   SEX M ☐ F ☐ | 4. INSURED'S NAME (Last Name, First Name, Middle Initial) |

| 5. PATIENT'S ADDRESS (No., Street) | 6. PATIENT RELATIONSHIP TO INSURED Self ☐ Spouse ☐ Child ☐ Other ☐ | 7. INSURED'S ADDRESS (No., Street) |

| CITY   STATE | 8. PATIENT STATUS Single ☐ Married ☐ Other ☐ | CITY   STATE |

| ZIP CODE   TELEPHONE (Include Area Code) (   ) | Employed ☐ Full-Time Student ☐ Part-Time Student ☐ | ZIP CODE   TELEPHONE (Include Area Code) (   ) |

| 9. OTHER INSURED'S NAME (Last Name, First Name, Middle Initial) | 10. IS PATIENT'S CONDITION RELATED TO: | 11. INSURED'S POLICY GROUP OR FECA NUMBER |

| a. OTHER INSURED'S POLICY OR GROUP NUMBER | a. EMPLOYMENT? (Current or Previous) YES ☐ NO ☐ | a. INSURED'S DATE OF BIRTH MM DD YY   SEX M ☐ F ☐ |

| b. OTHER INSURED'S DATE OF BIRTH MM DD YY   SEX M ☐ F ☐ | b. AUTO ACCIDENT?   PLACE (State) YES ☐ NO ☐ | b. EMPLOYER'S NAME OR SCHOOL NAME |

| c. EMPLOYER'S NAME OR SCHOOL NAME | c. OTHER ACCIDENT? YES ☐ NO ☐ | c. INSURANCE PLAN NAME OR PROGRAM NAME |

| d. INSURANCE PLAN NAME OR PROGRAM NAME | 10d. RESERVED FOR LOCAL USE | d. IS THERE ANOTHER HEALTH BENEFIT PLAN? YES ☐ NO ☐ If yes, return to and complete item 9 a-d. |

READ BACK OF FORM BEFORE COMPLETING & SIGNING THIS FORM.
12. PATIENT'S OR AUTHORIZED PERSON'S SIGNATURE I authorize the release of any medical or other information necessary to process this claim. I also request payment of government benefits either to myself or to the party who accepts assignment below.

SIGNED _____   DATE _____

13. INSURED'S OR AUTHORIZED PERSON'S SIGNATURE I authorize payment of medical benefits to the undersigned physician or supplier for services described below.

SIGNED _____

| 14. DATE OF CURRENT: MM DD YY ◄ ILLNESS (First symptom) OR INJURY (Accident) OR PREGNANCY(LMP) | 15. IF PATIENT HAS HAD SAME OR SIMILAR ILLNESS. GIVE FIRST DATE MM DD YY | 16. DATES PATIENT UNABLE TO WORK IN CURRENT OCCUPATION FROM MM DD YY   TO MM DD YY |

| 17. NAME OF REFERRING PROVIDER OR OTHER SOURCE | 17a. ___ 17b. NPI ___ | 18. HOSPITALIZATION DATES RELATED TO CURRENT SERVICES FROM MM DD YY   TO MM DD YY |

| 19. RESERVED FOR LOCAL USE | | 20. OUTSIDE LAB? YES ☐ NO ☐ $ CHARGES |

| 21. DIAGNOSIS OR NATURE OF ILLNESS OR INJURY (Relate Items 1, 2, 3 or 4 to Item 24E by Line) 1. L___.___   3. L___.___   2. L___.___   4. L___.___ | 22. MEDICAID RESUBMISSION CODE   ORIGINAL REF. NO. 23. PRIOR AUTHORIZATION NUMBER |

24. A. DATE(S) OF SERVICE From To MM DD YY MM DD YY	B. PLACE OF SERVICE	C. EMG	D. PROCEDURES, SERVICES, OR SUPPLIES (Explain Unusual Circumstances) CPT/HCPCS MODIFIER	E. DIAGNOSIS POINTER	F. $ CHARGES	G. DAYS OR UNITS	H. EPSDT Family Plan	I. ID. QUAL.	J. RENDERING PROVIDER ID. #
1									NPI
2									NPI
3									NPI
4									NPI
5									NPI
6									NPI

| 25. FEDERAL TAX I.D. NUMBER   SSN ☐ EIN ☐ | 26. PATIENT'S ACCOUNT NO. | 27. ACCEPT ASSIGNMENT? (For govt. claims, see back) YES ☐ NO ☐ | 28. TOTAL CHARGE $ | 29. AMOUNT PAID $ | 30. BALANCE DUE $ |

| 31. SIGNATURE OF PHYSICIAN OR SUPPLIER INCLUDING DEGREES OR CREDENTIALS (I certify that the statements on the reverse apply to this bill and are made a part thereof.) SIGNED _____ DATE _____ | 32. SERVICE FACILITY LOCATION INFORMATION a. NPI   b. | 33. BILLING PROVIDER INFO & PH # (123) 456-7890 DOUGLASVILLE MEDICINE ASSOCIATES 5076 BRAND BLVD, STE 401 DOUGLASVILLE, NY 01234 a. 9995010111   b. |

APPROVED OMB-0938-0999 FORM CMS-1500 (08/05)

CARRIER   PATIENT AND INSURED INFORMATION   PHYSICIAN OR SUPPLIER INFORMATION

1500

HEALTH INSURANCE CLAIM FORM

APPROVED BY NATIONAL UNIFORM CLAIM COMMITTEE 08/05

PICA		PICA

1. MEDICARE MEDICAID TRICARE CHAMPVA GROUP FECA OTHER CHAMPUS HEALTH PLAN BLK LUNG	1a. INSURED'S I.D. NUMBER (For Program in Item 1)
(Medicare #) (Medicaid #) (Sponsor's SSN) (Member ID#) (SSN or ID) (SSN) (ID)	

2. PATIENT'S NAME (Last Name, First Name, Middle Initial)

3. PATIENT'S BIRTH DATE MM DD YY **SEX** M ☐ F ☐

4. INSURED'S NAME (Last Name, First Name, Middle Initial)

5. PATIENT'S ADDRESS (No., Street)

6. PATIENT RELATIONSHIP TO INSURED Self ☐ Spouse ☐ Child ☐ Other ☐

7. INSURED'S ADDRESS (No., Street)

CITY STATE

8. PATIENT STATUS Single ☐ Married ☐ Other ☐

CITY STATE

ZIP CODE TELEPHONE (Include Area Code) ( )

Employed ☐ Full-Time Student ☐ Part-Time Student ☐

ZIP CODE TELEPHONE (Include Area Code) ( )

9. OTHER INSURED'S NAME (Last Name, First Name, Middle Initial)

10. IS PATIENT'S CONDITION RELATED TO:

11. INSURED'S POLICY GROUP OR FECA NUMBER

a. OTHER INSURED'S POLICY OR GROUP NUMBER

a. EMPLOYMENT? (Current or Previous) YES ☐ NO ☐

a. INSURED'S DATE OF BIRTH MM DD YY **SEX** M ☐ F ☐

b. OTHER INSURED'S DATE OF BIRTH MM DD YY **SEX** M ☐ F ☐

b. AUTO ACCIDENT? YES ☐ NO ☐ PLACE (State)

b. EMPLOYER'S NAME OR SCHOOL NAME

c. EMPLOYER'S NAME OR SCHOOL NAME

c. OTHER ACCIDENT? YES ☐ NO ☐

c. INSURANCE PLAN NAME OR PROGRAM NAME

d. INSURANCE PLAN NAME OR PROGRAM NAME

10d. RESERVED FOR LOCAL USE

d. IS THERE ANOTHER HEALTH BENEFIT PLAN? YES ☐ NO ☐ If yes, return to and complete item 9 a-d.

READ BACK OF FORM BEFORE COMPLETING & SIGNING THIS FORM.
12. PATIENT'S OR AUTHORIZED PERSON'S SIGNATURE I authorize the release of any medical or other information necessary to process this claim. I also request payment of government benefits either to myself or to the party who accepts assignment below.

SIGNED _____ DATE _____

13. INSURED'S OR AUTHORIZED PERSON'S SIGNATURE I authorize payment of medical benefits to the undersigned physician or supplier for services described below.

SIGNED _____

14. DATE OF CURRENT: MM DD YY ◄ ILLNESS (First symptom) OR INJURY (Accident) OR PREGNANCY(LMP)

15. IF PATIENT HAS HAD SAME OR SIMILAR ILLNESS. GIVE FIRST DATE MM DD YY

16. DATES PATIENT UNABLE TO WORK IN CURRENT OCCUPATION FROM MM DD YY TO MM DD YY

17. NAME OF REFERRING PROVIDER OR OTHER SOURCE

17a.
17b. NPI

18. HOSPITALIZATION DATES RELATED TO CURRENT SERVICES FROM MM DD YY TO MM DD YY

19. RESERVED FOR LOCAL USE

20. OUTSIDE LAB? YES ☐ NO ☐ $ CHARGES

21. DIAGNOSIS OR NATURE OF ILLNESS OR INJURY (Relate Items 1, 2, 3 or 4 to Item 24E by Line)

1. L___ . ___   3. L___ . ___
2. L___ . ___   4. L___ . ___

22. MEDICAID RESUBMISSION CODE ORIGINAL REF. NO.

23. PRIOR AUTHORIZATION NUMBER

24. A. DATE(S) OF SERVICE		B. PLACE OF SERVICE	C. EMG	D. PROCEDURES, SERVICES, OR SUPPLIES (Explain Unusual Circumstances)		E. DIAGNOSIS POINTER	F. $ CHARGES	G. DAYS OR UNITS	H. EPSDT Family Plan	I. ID. QUAL.	J. RENDERING PROVIDER ID. #
From MM DD YY	To MM DD YY			CPT/HCPCS	MODIFIER						
1										NPI	
2										NPI	
3										NPI	
4										NPI	
5										NPI	
6										NPI	

25. FEDERAL TAX I.D. NUMBER SSN ☐ EIN ☐

26. PATIENT'S ACCOUNT NO.

27. ACCEPT ASSIGNMENT? (For govt. claims, see back) YES ☐ NO ☐

28. TOTAL CHARGE $

29. AMOUNT PAID $

30. BALANCE DUE $

31. SIGNATURE OF PHYSICIAN OR SUPPLIER INCLUDING DEGREES OR CREDENTIALS (I certify that the statements on the reverse apply to this bill and are made a part thereof.)

SIGNED _____ DATE _____

32. SERVICE FACILITY LOCATION INFORMATION

a. NPI b.

33. BILLING PROVIDER INFO & PH # (123) 456-7890
DOUGLASVILLE MEDICINE ASSOCIATES
5076 BRAND BLVD, STE 401
DOUGLASVILLE, NY 01234
a. 9995010111 b.

NUCC Instruction Manual available at: www.nucc.org

APPROVED OMB-0938-0999 FORM CMS-1500 (08/05)

CARRIER

PATIENT AND INSURED INFORMATION

PHYSICIAN OR SUPPLIER INFORMATION

1500

HEALTH INSURANCE CLAIM FORM

APPROVED BY NATIONAL UNIFORM CLAIM COMMITTEE 08/05

☐☐ PICA | | PICA ☐☐

1. MEDICARE MEDICAID TRICARE CHAMPVA GROUP FECA OTHER | 1a. INSURED'S I.D. NUMBER (For Program in Item 1)
 CHAMPUS HEALTH PLAN BLK LUNG
 (Medicare #) (Medicaid #) (Sponsor's SSN) (Member ID#) (SSN or ID) (SSN) (ID)

2. PATIENT'S NAME (Last Name, First Name, Middle Initial) | 3. PATIENT'S BIRTH DATE   SEX | 4. INSURED'S NAME (Last Name, First Name, Middle Initial)
MM DD YY M ☐ F ☐

5. PATIENT'S ADDRESS (No., Street) | 6. PATIENT RELATIONSHIP TO INSURED | 7. INSURED'S ADDRESS (No., Street)
Self ☐ Spouse ☐ Child ☐ Other ☐

CITY | STATE | 8. PATIENT STATUS | CITY | STATE
Single ☐ Married ☐ Other ☐

ZIP CODE | TELEPHONE (Include Area Code) | Employed ☐ Full-Time Student ☐ Part-Time Student ☐ | ZIP CODE | TELEPHONE (Include Area Code)
( ) | | ( )

9. OTHER INSURED'S NAME (Last Name, First Name, Middle Initial) | 10. IS PATIENT'S CONDITION RELATED TO: | 11. INSURED'S POLICY GROUP OR FECA NUMBER

a. OTHER INSURED'S POLICY OR GROUP NUMBER | a. EMPLOYMENT? (Current or Previous) ☐ YES ☐ NO | a. INSURED'S DATE OF BIRTH SEX
MM DD YY M ☐ F ☐

b. OTHER INSURED'S DATE OF BIRTH SEX | b. AUTO ACCIDENT? PLACE (State) ☐ YES ☐ NO | b. EMPLOYER'S NAME OR SCHOOL NAME
MM DD YY M ☐ F ☐

c. EMPLOYER'S NAME OR SCHOOL NAME | c. OTHER ACCIDENT? ☐ YES ☐ NO | c. INSURANCE PLAN NAME OR PROGRAM NAME

d. INSURANCE PLAN NAME OR PROGRAM NAME | 10d. RESERVED FOR LOCAL USE | d. IS THERE ANOTHER HEALTH BENEFIT PLAN?
☐ YES ☐ NO If yes, return to and complete item 9 a-d.

READ BACK OF FORM BEFORE COMPLETING & SIGNING THIS FORM.
12. PATIENT'S OR AUTHORIZED PERSON'S SIGNATURE I authorize the release of any medical or other information necessary to process this claim. I also request payment of government benefits either to myself or to the party who accepts assignment below. | 13. INSURED'S OR AUTHORIZED PERSON'S SIGNATURE I authorize payment of medical benefits to the undersigned physician or supplier for services described below.

SIGNED _____ DATE _____ | SIGNED _____

14. DATE OF CURRENT: ☐ ILLNESS (First symptom) OR INJURY (Accident) OR PREGNANCY(LMP) | 15. IF PATIENT HAS HAD SAME OR SIMILAR ILLNESS. GIVE FIRST DATE MM DD YY | 16. DATES PATIENT UNABLE TO WORK IN CURRENT OCCUPATION
MM DD YY | FROM MM DD YY TO MM DD YY

17. NAME OF REFERRING PROVIDER OR OTHER SOURCE | 17a. | 18. HOSPITALIZATION DATES RELATED TO CURRENT SERVICES
17b. NPI | FROM MM DD YY TO MM DD YY

19. RESERVED FOR LOCAL USE | 20. OUTSIDE LAB? ☐ YES ☐ NO $ CHARGES

21. DIAGNOSIS OR NATURE OF ILLNESS OR INJURY (Relate Items 1, 2, 3 or 4 to Item 24E by Line) | 22. MEDICAID RESUBMISSION CODE ORIGINAL REF. NO.
1. |____.____| 3. |____.____| | 23. PRIOR AUTHORIZATION NUMBER
2. |____.____| 4. |____.____|

24. A. DATE(S) OF SERVICE						B. PLACE OF SERVICE	C. EMG	D. PROCEDURES, SERVICES, OR SUPPLIES (Explain Unusual Circumstances)		E. DIAGNOSIS POINTER	F. $ CHARGES	G. DAYS OR UNITS	H. EPSDT Family Plan	I. ID. QUAL.	J. RENDERING PROVIDER ID. #
From			To					CPT/HCPCS	MODIFIER						
MM	DD	YY	MM	DD	YY										
1														NPI	
2														NPI	
3														NPI	
4														NPI	
5														NPI	
6														NPI	

25. FEDERAL TAX I.D. NUMBER SSN ☐ EIN ☐ | 26. PATIENT'S ACCOUNT NO. | 27. ACCEPT ASSIGNMENT? (For govt. claims, see back) ☐ YES ☐ NO | 28. TOTAL CHARGE $ | 29. AMOUNT PAID $ | 30. BALANCE DUE $

31. SIGNATURE OF PHYSICIAN OR SUPPLIER INCLUDING DEGREES OR CREDENTIALS (I certify that the statements on the reverse apply to this bill and are made a part thereof.) | 32. SERVICE FACILITY LOCATION INFORMATION | 33. BILLING PROVIDER INFO & PH # (123) 456-7890
DOUGLASVILLE MEDICINE ASSOCIATES
5076 BRAND BLVD, STE 401
DOUGLASVILLE, NY 01234

SIGNED _____ DATE _____ | a. NPI   b. | a. 9995010111   b.

CARRIER

PATIENT AND INSURED INFORMATION

PHYSICIAN OR SUPPLIER INFORMATION

1500

HEALTH INSURANCE CLAIM FORM

APPROVED BY NATIONAL UNIFORM CLAIM COMMITTEE 08/05

☐☐☐ PICA | PICA ☐☐☐

| 1. MEDICARE ☐ (Medicare #) MEDICAID ☐ (Medicaid #) TRICARE CHAMPUS ☐ (Sponsor's SSN) CHAMPVA ☐ (Member ID#) GROUP HEALTH PLAN ☐ (SSN or ID) FECA BLK LUNG ☐ (SSN) OTHER ☐ (ID) | 1a. INSURED'S I.D. NUMBER | (For Program in Item 1) |

| 2. PATIENT'S NAME (Last Name, First Name, Middle Initial) | 3. PATIENT'S BIRTH DATE MM | DD | YY   SEX M ☐ F ☐ | 4. INSURED'S NAME (Last Name, First Name, Middle Initial) |

| 5. PATIENT'S ADDRESS (No., Street) | 6. PATIENT RELATIONSHIP TO INSURED Self ☐ Spouse ☐ Child ☐ Other ☐ | 7. INSURED'S ADDRESS (No., Street) |

| CITY | STATE | 8. PATIENT STATUS Single ☐ Married ☐ Other ☐ | CITY | STATE |

| ZIP CODE | TELEPHONE (Include Area Code) ( ) | Employed ☐ Full-Time Student ☐ Part-Time Student ☐ | ZIP CODE | TELEPHONE (Include Area Code) ( ) |

| 9. OTHER INSURED'S NAME (Last Name, First Name, Middle Initial) | 10. IS PATIENT'S CONDITION RELATED TO: | 11. INSURED'S POLICY GROUP OR FECA NUMBER |

| a. OTHER INSURED'S POLICY OR GROUP NUMBER | a. EMPLOYMENT? (Current or Previous) YES ☐ NO ☐ | a. INSURED'S DATE OF BIRTH MM | DD | YY   SEX M ☐ F ☐ |

| b. OTHER INSURED'S DATE OF BIRTH MM | DD | YY   SEX M ☐ F ☐ | b. AUTO ACCIDENT? PLACE (State) YES ☐ NO ☐ | b. EMPLOYER'S NAME OR SCHOOL NAME |

| c. EMPLOYER'S NAME OR SCHOOL NAME | c. OTHER ACCIDENT? YES ☐ NO ☐ | c. INSURANCE PLAN NAME OR PROGRAM NAME |

| d. INSURANCE PLAN NAME OR PROGRAM NAME | 10d. RESERVED FOR LOCAL USE | d. IS THERE ANOTHER HEALTH BENEFIT PLAN? YES ☐ NO ☐ If yes, return to and complete item 9 a-d. |

READ BACK OF FORM BEFORE COMPLETING & SIGNING THIS FORM.

12. PATIENT'S OR AUTHORIZED PERSON'S SIGNATURE I authorize the release of any medical or other information necessary to process this claim. I also request payment of government benefits either to myself or to the party who accepts assignment below.

SIGNED _____ DATE _____

13. INSURED'S OR AUTHORIZED PERSON'S SIGNATURE I authorize payment of medical benefits to the undersigned physician or supplier for services described below.

SIGNED _____

| 14. DATE OF CURRENT: MM | DD | YY ◄ ILLNESS (First symptom) OR INJURY (Accident) OR PREGNANCY(LMP) | 15. IF PATIENT HAS HAD SAME OR SIMILAR ILLNESS. GIVE FIRST DATE MM | DD | YY | 16. DATES PATIENT UNABLE TO WORK IN CURRENT OCCUPATION FROM MM | DD | YY   TO MM | DD | YY |

| 17. NAME OF REFERRING PROVIDER OR OTHER SOURCE | 17a. | 17b. NPI | 18. HOSPITALIZATION DATES RELATED TO CURRENT SERVICES FROM MM | DD | YY   TO MM | DD | YY |

| 19. RESERVED FOR LOCAL USE | 20. OUTSIDE LAB? YES ☐ NO ☐ | $ CHARGES |

21. DIAGNOSIS OR NATURE OF ILLNESS OR INJURY (Relate Items 1, 2, 3 or 4 to Item 24E by Line)

1. |___.___| 3. |___.___|

2. |___.___| 4. |___.___|

| 22. MEDICAID RESUBMISSION CODE | ORIGINAL REF. NO. |

23. PRIOR AUTHORIZATION NUMBER

24. A. DATE(S) OF SERVICE						B. PLACE OF SERVICE	C. EMG	D. PROCEDURES, SERVICES, OR SUPPLIES (Explain Unusual Circumstances) CPT/HCPCS	MODIFIER	E. DIAGNOSIS POINTER	F. $ CHARGES	G. DAYS OR UNITS	H. EPSDT Family Plan	I. ID. QUAL.	J. RENDERING PROVIDER ID. #
From MM	DD	YY	To MM	DD	YY										
1														NPI	
2														NPI	
3														NPI	
4														NPI	
5														NPI	
6														NPI	

| 25. FEDERAL TAX I.D. NUMBER SSN ☐ EIN ☐ | 26. PATIENT'S ACCOUNT NO. | 27. ACCEPT ASSIGNMENT? (For govt. claims, see back) YES ☐ NO ☐ | 28. TOTAL CHARGE $ | 29. AMOUNT PAID $ | 30. BALANCE DUE $ |

| 31. SIGNATURE OF PHYSICIAN OR SUPPLIER INCLUDING DEGREES OR CREDENTIALS (I certify that the statements on the reverse apply to this bill and are made a part thereof.) SIGNED _____ DATE _____ | 32. SERVICE FACILITY LOCATION INFORMATION a. NPI b. | 33. BILLING PROVIDER INFO & PH # (123) 456-7890 DOUGLASVILLE MEDICINE ASSOCIATES 5076 BRAND BLVD, STE 401 DOUGLASVILLE, NY 01234 a. 9995010111 b. |

NUCC Instruction Manual available at: www.nucc.org | APPROVED OMB-0938-0999 FORM CMS-1500 (08/05)

[1500]

HEALTH INSURANCE CLAIM FORM

APPROVED BY NATIONAL UNIFORM CLAIM COMMITTEE 08/05

☐☐ PICA   PICA ☐☐

1. MEDICARE	MEDICAID	TRICARE CHAMPUS	CHAMPVA	GROUP HEALTH PLAN	FECA BLK LUNG	OTHER	1a. INSURED'S I.D. NUMBER (For Program in Item 1)
☐ (Medicare #)	☐ (Medicaid #)	☐ (Sponsor's SSN)	☐ (Member ID#)	☐ (SSN or ID)	☐ (SSN)	☐ (ID)	

2. PATIENT'S NAME (Last Name, First Name, Middle Initial) | 3. PATIENT'S BIRTH DATE MM DD YY   SEX M☐ F☐ | 4. INSURED'S NAME (Last Name, First Name, Middle Initial)

5. PATIENT'S ADDRESS (No., Street) | 6. PATIENT RELATIONSHIP TO INSURED Self☐ Spouse☐ Child☐ Other☐ | 7. INSURED'S ADDRESS (No., Street)

CITY   STATE | 8. PATIENT STATUS Single☐ Married☐ Other☐ | CITY   STATE

ZIP CODE   TELEPHONE (Include Area Code) (   ) | Employed☐ Full-Time Student☐ Part-Time Student☐ | ZIP CODE   TELEPHONE (Include Area Code) (   )

9. OTHER INSURED'S NAME (Last Name, First Name, Middle Initial) | 10. IS PATIENT'S CONDITION RELATED TO: | 11. INSURED'S POLICY GROUP OR FECA NUMBER

a. OTHER INSURED'S POLICY OR GROUP NUMBER | a. EMPLOYMENT? (Current or Previous) ☐ YES ☐ NO | a. INSURED'S DATE OF BIRTH MM DD YY SEX M☐ F☐

b. OTHER INSURED'S DATE OF BIRTH MM DD YY SEX M☐ F☐ | b. AUTO ACCIDENT? PLACE (State) ☐ YES ☐ NO | b. EMPLOYER'S NAME OR SCHOOL NAME

c. EMPLOYER'S NAME OR SCHOOL NAME | c. OTHER ACCIDENT? ☐ YES ☐ NO | c. INSURANCE PLAN NAME OR PROGRAM NAME

d. INSURANCE PLAN NAME OR PROGRAM NAME | 10d. RESERVED FOR LOCAL USE | d. IS THERE ANOTHER HEALTH BENEFIT PLAN? ☐ YES ☐ NO *If yes,* return to and complete item 9 a-d.

READ BACK OF FORM BEFORE COMPLETING & SIGNING THIS FORM.

12. PATIENT'S OR AUTHORIZED PERSON'S SIGNATURE I authorize the release of any medical or other information necessary to process this claim. I also request payment of government benefits either to myself or to the party who accepts assignment below.

SIGNED _____   DATE _____

13. INSURED'S OR AUTHORIZED PERSON'S SIGNATURE I authorize payment of medical benefits to the undersigned physician or supplier for services described below.

SIGNED _____

14. DATE OF CURRENT: MM DD YY ◀ ILLNESS (First symptom) OR INJURY (Accident) OR PREGNANCY(LMP) | 15. IF PATIENT HAS HAD SAME OR SIMILAR ILLNESS. GIVE FIRST DATE MM DD YY | 16. DATES PATIENT UNABLE TO WORK IN CURRENT OCCUPATION FROM MM DD YY TO MM DD YY

17. NAME OF REFERRING PROVIDER OR OTHER SOURCE | 17a. ___ 17b. NPI ___ | 18. HOSPITALIZATION DATES RELATED TO CURRENT SERVICES FROM MM DD YY TO MM DD YY

19. RESERVED FOR LOCAL USE | 20. OUTSIDE LAB? ☐ YES ☐ NO $ CHARGES

21. DIAGNOSIS OR NATURE OF ILLNESS OR INJURY (Relate Items 1, 2, 3 or 4 to Item 24E by Line)
1. ⌊___.___⌋   3. ⌊___.___⌋
2. ⌊___.___⌋   4. ⌊___.___⌋

22. MEDICAID RESUBMISSION CODE   ORIGINAL REF. NO.

23. PRIOR AUTHORIZATION NUMBER

24. A. DATE(S) OF SERVICE From MM DD YY To MM DD YY	B. PLACE OF SERVICE	C. EMG	D. PROCEDURES, SERVICES, OR SUPPLIES (Explain Unusual Circumstances) CPT/HCPCS MODIFIER	E. DIAGNOSIS POINTER	F. $ CHARGES	G. DAYS OR UNITS	H. EPSDT Family Plan	I. ID. QUAL.	J. RENDERING PROVIDER ID. #
1								NPI	
2								NPI	
3								NPI	
4								NPI	
5								NPI	
6								NPI	

25. FEDERAL TAX I.D. NUMBER ☐ SSN ☐ EIN | 26. PATIENT'S ACCOUNT NO. | 27. ACCEPT ASSIGNMENT? (For govt. claims, see back) ☐ YES ☐ NO | 28. TOTAL CHARGE $ | 29. AMOUNT PAID $ | 30. BALANCE DUE $

31. SIGNATURE OF PHYSICIAN OR SUPPLIER INCLUDING DEGREES OR CREDENTIALS (I certify that the statements on the reverse apply to this bill and are made a part thereof.)

SIGNED _____   DATE _____

32. SERVICE FACILITY LOCATION INFORMATION

a. NPI   b.

33. BILLING PROVIDER INFO & PH # (123) 456-7890
DOUGLASVILLE MEDICINE ASSOCIATES
5076 BRAND BLVD, STE 401
DOUGLASVILLE, NY 01234
a. 9995010111   b.

NUCC Instruction Manual available at: www.nucc.org   APPROVED OMB-0938-0999 FORM CMS-1500 (08/05)

Right margin vertical text: CARRIER → | ← PATIENT AND INSURED INFORMATION → | ← PHYSICIAN OR SUPPLIER INFORMATION →

1500

HEALTH INSURANCE CLAIM FORM

APPROVED BY NATIONAL UNIFORM CLAIM COMMITTEE 08/05

☐☐☐ PICA | PICA ☐☐☐

| 1. MEDICARE MEDICAID TRICARE CHAMPUS CHAMPVA GROUP HEALTH PLAN FECA BLK LUNG OTHER | 1a. INSURED'S I.D. NUMBER (For Program in Item 1) |

1. ☐ (Medicare #) ☐ (Medicaid #) ☐ (Sponsor's SSN) ☐ (Member ID#) ☐ (SSN or ID) ☐ (SSN) ☐ (ID)

2. PATIENT'S NAME (Last Name, First Name, Middle Initial)

3. PATIENT'S BIRTH DATE SEX
MM DD YY M ☐ F ☐

4. INSURED'S NAME (Last Name, First Name, Middle Initial)

5. PATIENT'S ADDRESS (No., Street)

6. PATIENT RELATIONSHIP TO INSURED
Self ☐ Spouse ☐ Child ☐ Other ☐

7. INSURED'S ADDRESS (No., Street)

CITY   STATE

8. PATIENT STATUS
Single ☐ Married ☐ Other ☐

CITY   STATE

ZIP CODE   TELEPHONE (Include Area Code)
(   )

Employed ☐ Full-Time Student ☐ Part-Time Student ☐

ZIP CODE   TELEPHONE (Include Area Code)
(   )

9. OTHER INSURED'S NAME (Last Name, First Name, Middle Initial)

10. IS PATIENT'S CONDITION RELATED TO:

11. INSURED'S POLICY GROUP OR FECA NUMBER

a. OTHER INSURED'S POLICY OR GROUP NUMBER

a. EMPLOYMENT? (Current or Previous)
☐ YES ☐ NO

a. INSURED'S DATE OF BIRTH SEX
MM DD YY M ☐ F ☐

b. OTHER INSURED'S DATE OF BIRTH SEX
MM DD YY M ☐ F ☐

b. AUTO ACCIDENT?   PLACE (State)
☐ YES ☐ NO

b. EMPLOYER'S NAME OR SCHOOL NAME

c. EMPLOYER'S NAME OR SCHOOL NAME

c. OTHER ACCIDENT?
☐ YES ☐ NO

c. INSURANCE PLAN NAME OR PROGRAM NAME

d. INSURANCE PLAN NAME OR PROGRAM NAME

10d. RESERVED FOR LOCAL USE

d. IS THERE ANOTHER HEALTH BENEFIT PLAN?
☐ YES ☐ NO *If yes*, return to and complete item 9 a-d.

READ BACK OF FORM BEFORE COMPLETING & SIGNING THIS FORM.

12. PATIENT'S OR AUTHORIZED PERSON'S SIGNATURE I authorize the release of any medical or other information necessary to process this claim. I also request payment of government benefits either to myself or to the party who accepts assignment below.

SIGNED _____ DATE _____

13. INSURED'S OR AUTHORIZED PERSON'S SIGNATURE I authorize payment of medical benefits to the undersigned physician or supplier for services described below.

SIGNED _____

14. DATE OF CURRENT: ◄ ILLNESS (First symptom) OR
MM DD YY   INJURY (Accident) OR
                PREGNANCY(LMP)

15. IF PATIENT HAS HAD SAME OR SIMILAR ILLNESS.
GIVE FIRST DATE MM DD YY

16. DATES PATIENT UNABLE TO WORK IN CURRENT OCCUPATION
FROM MM DD YY TO MM DD YY

17. NAME OF REFERRING PROVIDER OR OTHER SOURCE

17a.
17b. NPI

18. HOSPITALIZATION DATES RELATED TO CURRENT SERVICES
FROM MM DD YY TO MM DD YY

19. RESERVED FOR LOCAL USE

20. OUTSIDE LAB? $ CHARGES
☐ YES ☐ NO

21. DIAGNOSIS OR NATURE OF ILLNESS OR INJURY (Relate Items 1, 2, 3 or 4 to Item 24E by Line)

1. └___ . ___   3. └___ . ___

2. └___ . ___   4. └___ . ___

22. MEDICAID RESUBMISSION CODE   ORIGINAL REF. NO.

23. PRIOR AUTHORIZATION NUMBER

24. A. DATE(S) OF SERVICE		B. PLACE OF SERVICE	C. EMG	D. PROCEDURES, SERVICES, OR SUPPLIES (Explain Unusual Circumstances) CPT/HCPCS MODIFIER	E. DIAGNOSIS POINTER	F. $ CHARGES	G. DAYS OR UNITS	H. EPSDT Family Plan	I. ID. QUAL.	J. RENDERING PROVIDER ID. #
From To										
MM DD YY MM DD YY										
1									NPI	
2									NPI	
3									NPI	
4									NPI	
5									NPI	
6									NPI	

25. FEDERAL TAX I.D. NUMBER SSN EIN ☐☐

26. PATIENT'S ACCOUNT NO.

27. ACCEPT ASSIGNMENT? (For govt. claims, see back)
☐ YES ☐ NO

28. TOTAL CHARGE
$

29. AMOUNT PAID
$

30. BALANCE DUE
$

31. SIGNATURE OF PHYSICIAN OR SUPPLIER INCLUDING DEGREES OR CREDENTIALS
(I certify that the statements on the reverse apply to this bill and are made a part thereof.)

SIGNED _____ DATE _____

32. SERVICE FACILITY LOCATION INFORMATION

a. NPI b.

33. BILLING PROVIDER INFO & PH # (123) 456-7890
DOUGLASVILLE MEDICINE ASSOCIATES
5076 BRAND BLVD, STE 401
DOUGLASVILLE, NY 01234
a. 9995010111 b.

NUCC Instruction Manual available at: www.nucc.org

APPROVED OMB-0938-0999 FORM CMS-1500 (08/05)

1500

HEALTH INSURANCE CLAIM FORM

APPROVED BY NATIONAL UNIFORM CLAIM COMMITTEE 08/05

PICA		PICA

1. MEDICARE ☐ (Medicare #) MEDICAID ☐ (Medicaid #) TRICARE CHAMPUS ☐ (Sponsor's SSN) CHAMPVA ☐ (Member ID#) GROUP HEALTH PLAN ☐ (SSN or ID) FECA BLK LUNG ☐ (SSN) OTHER ☐ (ID)	1a. INSURED'S I.D. NUMBER (For Program in Item 1)

2. PATIENT'S NAME (Last Name, First Name, Middle Initial)

3. PATIENT'S BIRTH DATE MM | DD | YY   SEX M ☐ F ☐

4. INSURED'S NAME (Last Name, First Name, Middle Initial)

5. PATIENT'S ADDRESS (No., Street)

6. PATIENT RELATIONSHIP TO INSURED Self ☐ Spouse ☐ Child ☐ Other ☐

7. INSURED'S ADDRESS (No., Street)

CITY   STATE

8. PATIENT STATUS Single ☐ Married ☐ Other ☐ Employed ☐ Full-Time Student ☐ Part-Time Student ☐

CITY   STATE

ZIP CODE   TELEPHONE (Include Area Code) (   )

ZIP CODE   TELEPHONE (Include Area Code) (   )

9. OTHER INSURED'S NAME (Last Name, First Name, Middle Initial)

10. IS PATIENT'S CONDITION RELATED TO:

11. INSURED'S POLICY GROUP OR FECA NUMBER

a. OTHER INSURED'S POLICY OR GROUP NUMBER

a. EMPLOYMENT? (Current or Previous) ☐ YES ☐ NO

a. INSURED'S DATE OF BIRTH MM | DD | YY   SEX M ☐ F ☐

b. OTHER INSURED'S DATE OF BIRTH MM | DD | YY   SEX M ☐ F ☐

b. AUTO ACCIDENT?   PLACE (State) ☐ YES ☐ NO

b. EMPLOYER'S NAME OR SCHOOL NAME

c. EMPLOYER'S NAME OR SCHOOL NAME

c. OTHER ACCIDENT? ☐ YES ☐ NO

c. INSURANCE PLAN NAME OR PROGRAM NAME

d. INSURANCE PLAN NAME OR PROGRAM NAME

10d. RESERVED FOR LOCAL USE

d. IS THERE ANOTHER HEALTH BENEFIT PLAN? ☐ YES ☐ NO   *If yes,* return to and complete item 9 a-d.

READ BACK OF FORM BEFORE COMPLETING & SIGNING THIS FORM.
12. PATIENT'S OR AUTHORIZED PERSON'S SIGNATURE I authorize the release of any medical or other information necessary to process this claim. I also request payment of government benefits either to myself or to the party who accepts assignment below.

SIGNED _____   DATE _____

13. INSURED'S OR AUTHORIZED PERSON'S SIGNATURE I authorize payment of medical benefits to the undersigned physician or supplier for services described below.

SIGNED _____

14. DATE OF CURRENT: MM | DD | YY ◄ ILLNESS (First symptom) OR INJURY (Accident) OR PREGNANCY(LMP)

15. IF PATIENT HAS HAD SAME OR SIMILAR ILLNESS. GIVE FIRST DATE MM | DD | YY

16. DATES PATIENT UNABLE TO WORK IN CURRENT OCCUPATION FROM MM | DD | YY TO MM | DD | YY

17. NAME OF REFERRING PROVIDER OR OTHER SOURCE

17a.
17b. NPI

18. HOSPITALIZATION DATES RELATED TO CURRENT SERVICES FROM MM | DD | YY TO MM | DD | YY

19. RESERVED FOR LOCAL USE

20. OUTSIDE LAB? ☐ YES ☐ NO $ CHARGES

21. DIAGNOSIS OR NATURE OF ILLNESS OR INJURY (Relate Items 1, 2, 3 or 4 to Item 24E by Line)

1. L___ . ___

3. L___ . ___

2. L___ . ___

4. L___ . ___

22. MEDICAID RESUBMISSION CODE   ORIGINAL REF. NO.

23. PRIOR AUTHORIZATION NUMBER

24. A. DATE(S) OF SERVICE From MM DD YY To MM DD YY	B. PLACE OF SERVICE	C. EMG	D. PROCEDURES, SERVICES, OR SUPPLIES (Explain Unusual Circumstances) CPT/HCPCS	MODIFIER	E. DIAGNOSIS POINTER	F. $ CHARGES	G. DAYS OR UNITS	H. EPSDT Family Plan	I. ID. QUAL.	J. RENDERING PROVIDER ID. #
1									NPI	
2									NPI	
3									NPI	
4									NPI	
5									NPI	
6									NPI	

25. FEDERAL TAX I.D. NUMBER ☐ SSN ☐ EIN

26. PATIENT'S ACCOUNT NO.

27. ACCEPT ASSIGNMENT? (For govt. claims, see back) ☐ YES ☐ NO

28. TOTAL CHARGE $

29. AMOUNT PAID $

30. BALANCE DUE $

31. SIGNATURE OF PHYSICIAN OR SUPPLIER INCLUDING DEGREES OR CREDENTIALS (I certify that the statements on the reverse apply to this bill and are made a part thereof.)

SIGNED _____ DATE _____

32. SERVICE FACILITY LOCATION INFORMATION

a. NPI   b.

33. BILLING PROVIDER INFO & PH # (123) 456-7890

DOUGLASVILLE MEDICINE ASSOCIATES
5076 BRAND BLVD, STE 401
DOUGLASVILLE, NY 01234

a. 9995010111   b.

NUCC Instruction Manual available at: www.nucc.org

APPROVED OMB-0938-0999 FORM CMS-1500 (08/05)

DEPOSIT TICKET

TO INSURE CLEAR COPY PRESS FIRMLY ON PEN
USE THIS TICKET FOR ALL DEPOSITS ENDORSE ALL CHECKS
WHEN MAILING DEPOSIT, PLEASE PRINT OR TYPE ADDRESS

DATE

	DOLLARS	CENTS
BILLS		
COIN		
CHECKS 1		
2		
3		
4		
5		
6		
7		
8		
9		
10		
11		
12		
13		
14		
15		
16		
17		
18		
19		
20		
TOTAL		

FOR INSTRUCTIONAL USE ONLY

L.D. HEATH, M.D.
4076 Brand Blvd., ste 401
Douglasville, NY 01234

THE FIRST NATIONAL BANK
Douglasville, NY

⑆0⒊⒑000059⑈ ⒈⒉0⼂⼂9⒈6 ⒊⼂⼂

3-2
310

FOR
BANK USE

CHECKS AND OTHER ITEMS ARE RECIEVED FOR DEPOSIT
SUBJECT TO THE PROVISIONS OF THE UNIFORM COMMERCIAL
CODE OR ANY APPLICABLE COLLECTION AGREEMENT

DEPOSIT TICKET

TO INSURE CLEAR COPY PRESS FIRMLY ON PEN
USE THIS TICKET FOR ALL DEPOSITS ENDORSE ALL CHECKS
WHEN MAILING DEPOSIT, PLEASE PRINT OR TYPE ADDRESS

DATE

	DOLLARS	CENTS
BILLS		
COIN		
CHECKS 1		
2		
3		
4		
5		
6		
7		
8		
9		
10		
11		
12		
13		
14		
15		
16		
17		
18		
19		
20		
TOTAL		

FOR INSTRUCTIONAL USE ONLY

L.D. HEATH, M.D.
4076 Brand Blvd., ste 401
Douglasville, NY 01234

THE FIRST NATIONAL BANK
Douglasville, NY

⑆0⒊⒑000059⑈ ⒈⒉0⼂⼂9⒈6 ⒊⼂⼂

3-2
310

FOR
BANK USE

CHECKS AND OTHER ITEMS ARE RECIEVED FOR DEPOSIT
SUBJECT TO THE PROVISIONS OF THE UNIFORM COMMERCIAL
CODE OR ANY APPLICABLE COLLECTION AGREEMENT

DEPOSIT TICKET

TO INSURE CLEAR COPY PRESS FIRMLY ON PEN
USE THIS TICKET FOR ALL DEPOSITS ENDORSE ALL CHECKS
WHEN MAILING DEPOSIT, PLEASE PRINT OR TYPE ADDRESS

DATE

		DOLLARS	CENTS
BILLS			
COIN			
CHECKS	1		
	2		
	3		
	4		
	5		
	6		
	7		
	8		
	9		
	10		
	11		
	12		
	13		
	14		
	15		
	16		
	17		
	18		
	19		
	20		
TOTAL			

FOR INSTRUCTIONAL USE ONLY

L.D. HEATH, M.D.
4076 Brand Blvd., ste 401
Douglasville, NY 01234

THE FIRST NATIONAL BANK
Douglasville, NY

⑈031⑈0000 59⑈: ⑈70ꞏꞏꞏ9⑈6   3⑈ꞏ

3-2
310

FOR
BANK USE

CHECKS AND OTHER ITEMS ARE RECIEVED FOR DEPOSIT
SUBJECT TO THE PROVISIONS OF THE UNIFORM COMMERCIAL
CODE OR ANY APPLICABLE COLLECTION AGREEMENT

DEPOSIT TICKET

TO INSURE CLEAR COPY PRESS FIRMLY ON PEN
USE THIS TICKET FOR ALL DEPOSITS ENDORSE ALL CHECKS
WHEN MAILING DEPOSIT, PLEASE PRINT OR TYPE ADDRESS

DATE

		DOLLARS	CENTS
BILLS			
COIN			
CHECKS	1		
	2		
	3		
	4		
	5		
	6		
	7		
	8		
	9		
	10		
	11		
	12		
	13		
	14		
	15		
	16		
	17		
	18		
	19		
	20		
TOTAL			

FOR INSTRUCTIONAL USE ONLY

L.D. HEATH, M.D.
4076 Brand Blvd., ste 401
Douglasville, NY 01234

THE FIRST NATIONAL BANK
Douglasville, NY

⑈031⑈0000 59⑈: ⑈70ꞏꞏꞏ9⑈6   3⑈ꞏ

3-2
310

FOR
BANK USE

CHECKS AND OTHER ITEMS ARE RECIEVED FOR DEPOSIT
SUBJECT TO THE PROVISIONS OF THE UNIFORM COMMERCIAL
CODE OR ANY APPLICABLE COLLECTION AGREEMENT

DEPOSIT TICKET

TO INSURE CLEAR COPY <u>PRESS FIRMLY ON PEN</u>
USE THIS TICKET FOR ALL DEPOSITS ENDORSE ALL CHECKS
WHEN MAILING DEPOSIT, PLEASE <u>PRINT OR TYPE</u> ADDRESS

DATE

L.D. HEATH, M.D.
4076 Brand Blvd., ste 401
Douglasville, NY 01234

FOR INSTRUCTIONAL USE ONLY

THE FIRST NATIONAL BANK
Douglasville, NY

⑆031000059⑆: ⑈70⑆916 ⑆3⑆

3-2
310

	DOLLARS	CENTS
BILLS		
COIN		
CHECKS 1		
2		
3		
4		
5		
6		
7		
8		
9		
10		
11		
12		
13		
14		
15		
16		
17		
18		
19		
20		
TOTAL		

FOR
BANK USE

CHECKS AND OTHER ITEMS ARE RECIEVED FOR DEPOSIT
SUBJECT TO THE PROVISIONS OF THE UNIFORM COMMERCIAL
CODE OR ANY APPLICABLE COLLECTION AGREEMENT

Name: _____

Date: _____

Approved: _____

DAILY CHECKUP: MONDAY, MARCH 4

1. What time was Walter Adams's appointment today? _____

2. What is the number of Pamela Cameron's receipt? _____

3. What is the name of Walter Adams's insurance company? _____

4. What is the balance of Maureen Michaels's account? _____

5. What is the cost of three boxes of TB syringes? _____

6. What is the diagnosis for Michele McLoud? _____

7. How often does Raymond O'Neill see Dr. Heath? _____

8. What is the charge for blood handling? _____

9. What is the ICD-9 code for benign hypertension? _____

10. Where does Pamela Cameron work? _____

11. What is the amount of total accounts receivable as of the end of today? _____

12. What diagnostic procedure did Walter Adams have done in the office today? _____

13. Which patient cancelled an appointment today? _____

14. What is this page's Column C total on the day sheet? _____

15. What is the fee for a hematocrit? _____

16. What is the balance on Michele McLoud's account? _____

17. To whom is check No. 480 written? _____

18. Will Dr. Heath accept budget payments? _____

19. What is the total of month-to-date adjustments? _____

20. What is the telephone number for Christopher Likens? _____

Name: _____

Date: _____

Approved: _____

DAILY CHECKUP: TUESDAY, MARCH 5

1. What was the payment amount received from Signal HMO for Alan Silverstein? _____

2. What is Anna Miller's balance as of the end of today? _____

3. On the day sheet, in which column of the Business Analysis Summaries is a chest x-ray recorded? _____

4. What is the charge for Tracey Mascello's office visit? _____

5. What is the total amount of payments collected in cash today? _____

6. What was the purpose of check No. 481 for $200? _____

7. What are the CPT codes for Tracey Mascello's visit today? _____

8. Which patient had a refund posted on the day sheet? _____

9. What is Elena Blanco's telephone number? _____

10. What is the amount of the total deposit for today? _____

11. Which patient was a "no-show" today? _____

12. Which patient cancelled an appointment today? _____

13. How many entries are posted on the day sheet today? _____

14. What are the total charges for today? _____

15. What is Christopher Likens's diagnosis? _____

16. When was Mary McDonald hospitalized? _____

17. What is the ICD-9 code for acute bronchitis? _____

18. What is the monthly service charge for City Answering Service? _____

19. What is another name for Column B-1 on the day sheet? _____

20. What type of insurance does Christopher Likens carry? _____

Name: _____

Date: _____

Approved: _____

DAILY CHECKUP: WEDNESDAY, MARCH 6

1. What is the name of Pamela Cameron's insurance company? _____

2. What is the balance of Jordan Connell's account as of the end of today? _____

3. What is the amount of state withholding tax for Joseph Pinelli? _____

4. What is the amount withheld from Sara Jackson's paycheck for Medicare? _____

5. How many superbills were given out today? _____

6. What is the amount of the total deposit for today? _____

7. What is the name of the firm for which Margaret Chandler works? _____

8. What are the total charges as of the end of today? _____

9. What is the ICD-CM code for angina pectoris, unspecified? _____

10. What is Eric Garcia's Social Security number? _____

11. What is the amount of the check received from Medicare Statewide Insurance Company? _____

12. Why was cash paid out today? _____

13. What time did Dr. Heath reserve for emergency visits today? _____

14. What is Raymond O'Neill's telephone number? _____

15. What time is Pamela Cameron's appointment tomorrow? _____

16. What is today's total in Column D on the day sheet? _____

17. Who is Dolores Perez's insurance carrier? _____

18. How many people are on the patient list for tomorrow? _____

19. What is the month-to-date current balance for today? _____

20. What is the bank balance as of the end of today (including today's deposit)? _____

DAILY CHECKUP: THURSDAY, MARCH 7

1. What is the amount of the invoice from Doctors' Medical Supply? _____

2. What is the current balance of Susan Deng's account? _____

3. What two appointment slots did Dr. Heath set aside for emergencies today? _____

4. What is the cash deposit today? _____

5. What is Eric Garcia's insurance group number? _____

6. What two procedure codes apply to Eric Garcia's visit? _____

7. What is the bank balance as of the end of today (including today's deposit)? _____

8. Which patient needed to be taken to the hospital by ambulance today? _____

9. How much cash is on hand at the beginning of the day? _____

10. What is the amount of check No. 486? _____

11. What is the amount of Margaret Chandler's copayment? _____

12. Which patient wrote a check for $50 to Dr. Heath? _____

13. What is the current balance of Deanna Hartsfeld's account? _____

14. When is Raymond O'Neill's next appointment? _____

15. What is the current balance of Pamela Cameron's account? _____

16. What is the procedure code for a glucose test? _____

17. What is the cost of six bottles of EKG gel? _____

18. What is the total accounts receivable as of the end of today? _____

19. What is the ICD-9 code for diabetes mellitus type 2, (non-insulin-dependent)? _____

20. What is the number of the receipt for Walter Adams? _____

Name: _____

Date: _____

Approved: _____

DAILY CHECKUP: FRIDAY, MARCH 8

1. What is Megan Caldwell's diagnosis? _____

2. What was the bank deposit for today? _____

3. What was the amount of the account payable for Englewood Accounting Services? _____

4. What was the number of Andrew Jefferson's receipt? _____

5. What were the charges for Bryan Lake? _____

6. What were the total charges for today? _____

7. What is the balance of Anna Miller's bill? _____

8. What was the amount Medicaid paid for Christopher Likens? _____

9. Who was given receipt No. 162? _____

10. What is the procedure code for an EKG? _____

11. What is the total amount of payments collected in cash today? _____

12. What was the charge for Bryan Lake's last appointment? _____

13. What does UTI stand for? _____

14. Which patient account received a payment from a collection agency today? _____

15. What is the name of Helen Baldwin's nearest relative? _____

16. Where is Mary McDonald employed? _____

17. What is the charge for a urinalysis? _____

18. What is the ICD-CM code for GERD? _____

19. How much are the charges for laboratory fees today? _____

20. How many entries were posted to today's day sheet? _____

Name: _____

Date: _____

Approved: _____

SECTION 2 WEEKLY CHECKUP: MARCH 4–8

1. Prepare a Schedule of Accounts Receivable, as of the end of the workday, March 8, showing the name of each patient and the current balance of his or her account (list names in alphabetical order):

Patient's Name	Current Balance	Patient's Name	Current Balance
_____	_____	_____	_____
_____	_____	_____	_____
_____	_____	_____	_____
_____	_____	_____	_____
_____	_____	_____	_____
_____	_____	_____	_____
_____	_____	_____	_____
_____	_____	_____	_____
_____	_____	_____	_____
_____	_____	_____	_____
_____	_____	_____	_____
_____	_____	_____	_____
_____	_____	_____	_____
_____	_____	_____	_____
_____	_____	_____	_____

Total Balance Due: _____

Note: The Total Accounts Receivable shown above will not agree with the Total Accounts Receivable shown on day sheet No. 47 because this simulation does not contain all of Dr. Heath's ledger cards.

2. From your completed day sheet No. 47, record the following information:

Month-to-date Payments _____

Month-to-date Adjustments _____

Total Accounts Receivable _____

Total Deposit _____

Closing Cash on Hand _____

3. From your completed check register, record the following totals in dollar amounts:

Checks Written	_____	Deposits	_____
Medical Supplies	_____	Rent Expense	_____
Utilities Expense	_____	Telephone Expense	_____
Office Supplies	_____	Fed. Withholding	_____
Books and Journals	_____	State Withholding	_____
Dues and Meetings	_____	SS and Medicare	_____
Cleaning Expense	_____	Net Payroll	_____
Insurance Expense	_____	Miscellaneous	_____
Maint. and Repairs	_____		

4. Complete this chart of the Business Analysis Summaries for the week in dollar amounts.

Date	Office Visits	Hospital Visits	Laboratory	Diagnostic	Injections	Misc.
TOTALS						

SECTION 3 WEEKLY CHECKUP: MARCH 4–8

1. What is Nancy Herbert's new address? _____

2. What type of secondary insurance does Xao Chang have? _____

3. What did Josephine Albertson change her name to? _____

4. What time is Mr. Chang's appointment on March 7, 2013? _____

5. What is Nancy Herbert's diagnosis? _____

6. How many minutes were allowed for Jordan Connell's physical? _____

7. On the Patient Appointment Form, in Field 9: Status, what is the meaning of R6? _____

8. What patients are listed on the Insurance Prebilling Worksheet? _____

9. What CPT code was listed for Andrew Jefferson on March 8? _____

10. What is Deanna Hartsfeld's husband's name? _____

11. Which three physician names are listed on the appointment calendar? _____

12. How many minutes were scheduled for hospital rounds on March 4 and March 18? _____

13. What day of the week was the Staff Breakfast scheduled? _____

14. Which two patients entered as new patients in the pegboard system were added as new patients to the MOSS computer system? _____

15. Which patient changed physicians from Dr. Schwartz to Dr. Heath? _____

16. What is the address of Signal HMO? _____

17. What does the Aging Report by Insurance Carriers show? _____

18. What is the fax number and website for Douglasville Medicine Associates? _____

19. What type of practice is Douglasville Medicine Associates? _____

20. What three criteria may be used to locate patients within the MOSS system? _____